W9-CIB-616

610.92 Goldm

Goldman, B.
The night shift.

MAY 07 2011

PRICE: $29.99 (3559/hc   )

THE NIGHT SHIFT

THE
NIGHT
SHIFT

REAL LIFE IN THE HEART OF THE E.R.

DR. BRIAN GOLDMAN

HarperCollins*Publishers*Ltd

The Night Shift
Copyright © 2010 by Brian Goldman Enterprises Ltd.
All rights reserved.

Published by HarperCollins Publishers Ltd

First Canadian edition

No part of this book may be used or reproduced in any manner
whatsoever without the prior written permission of the publisher,
except in the case of brief quotations embodied in reviews.

This book endeavours to be as true as possible to the author's real-life experience
in emergency medicine. Patients as they appear in the book are not actual people;
the author has drawn on real patient encounters throughout his career.
This book does not provide medical advice.

The views in this work are the author's own and do
not necessarily represent the views of Mount Sinai Hospital.

HarperCollins books may be purchased for educational, business,
or sales promotional use through our Special Markets Department.

HarperCollins Publishers Ltd
2 Bloor Street East, 20th Floor
Toronto, Ontario, Canada
M4W 1A8

www.harpercollins.ca

Library and Archives Canada Cataloguing in Publication

Goldman, Brian, 1956–
The night shift : real life in the heart of the E.R. / Brian Goldman.

ISBN 978-1-55468-391-8

1. Goldman, Brian, 1956–. 2. Hospitals—Emergency service.
3. Emergency physicians—Canada—Biography. I. Title.
RA975.5.E5G64 2010   610.92   C2010-903042-7

Printed and bound in the United States

RRD   9 8 7 6 5 4 3 2 1

To my partner, Tamara,
my children, Kaille and Sasha,
and to the thousands of patients who have
placed their trust in me

CONTENTS

ACKNOWLEDGEMENTS

This book would not have been possible without the support of Dr. Howard Ovens, my boss and the director of the Schwartz-Reisman Emergency Centre at Mount Sinai Hospital. Howard has been a friend, co-worker and mentor since I arrived at the hospital in 1984.

I want to celebrate an incredibly talented and dedicated group of fellow emergency physicians. To Howard, Bjug, Dave, Shirley, Tom, Sev; Yasmine, Shauna, John, Erin, Cheryl, Luke, Don, Mike, Ian, Harold, Howie and Jeff: thank you for sharing your stories, for sharing the burden of working nights, and for taking care of my patients when it's time for me to go home. To Evan, thank you for taking on the thankless task of working permanently on weekend nights.

When I work nights, I'm the only physician on duty. My real night companions are the many nurses, service assistants and others I've had the pleasure of working with the past twenty-five years. To Linda, Jackie, Josie, Gaye, Kaarlyn, Laura, Vince, Dolores, Evelyn, Don,

Behnaz, Terry, Emmett, Dave, Grant, Amy, Arianna, Emily, Kate, Lisa, Quinn, Lesley, Erin, Anna, Sonia, Allison, Vlad and many, many others: thank you for your hard work and your jokes, and for helping create the culture of the night shift I have come to know and love.

A big thank you also goes to Joseph Mapa, the president and CEO of Mount Sinai Hospital, for placing his support behind my efforts to bring my radio show to life and for running a fine hospital.

The ER at Mount Sinai Hospital is a busy place. Still, we don't see a lot of blood and guts on an average night. For this reason, I interviewed colleagues in emergency medicine from across Canada with stories to tell. Thank you to Drs. Ronald Stewart, Bruce Campana, David Lendrum, Stephen Friedman, Eddy Lang and Pat Croskerry for sharing your memories. Thanks goes to writer Sam Solomon, who conducted some of those interviews.

In particular, I want to single out Dr. Bruce Campana, whose courage, candour and storytelling on *White Coat, Black Art* and in this book have been an inspiration to me.

I owe a tremendous debt of gratitude to my friends and colleagues at the Canadian Broadcasting Corporation, who helped support and nurture my radio show *White Coat, Black Art*. I want to thank Ramona Dearing and Stewart Young, who were among the show's first champions on CBC Radio's program development committee. I want to thank producers Laura Carlin, Carma Jolly, Lara Hindle and Dominic Girard for their talent and contributions. I want to thank Talin Vartanian for producing the show's first season, which aired during the summer of 2007. In particular, I want to single out Quade Hermann for helping develop the original concept of the show, for producing the pilot episode and for being the show's producer during the past three seasons, during which *White Coat, Black Art* found its voice and its audience.

I want to thank Linda Groen, executive producer for radio current affairs, and Chris Boyce, CBC Radio's director of programming, for their incredible support.

I'd like to thank the doctors, nurses and other health professionals whose voices have made their way into the pages of this book via *White Coat, Black Art,* and also CBC for its permission to use the material here.

At HarperCollins, I am extremely grateful to my editor, Jim Gifford, who has an incredible gift for nurturing new book writers like me through the process. Thanks as well to production editor Allegra Robinson for catching my many doctorly errors in style and syntax. To CEO David Kent, thank you for sharing my passion for the world of medicine. You would have made a fine physician.

To my agent, Rick Broadhead, thanks for sticking with me through a long journey that started with a proposal for a book that turned into a radio series and then back into a book!

This book would not be possible without the Herculean efforts of writer and braodcaster Paul McLaughlin, who shepherded me through the myriad details of researching, organizing, writing and editing of this book.

To my partner, Tamara, thanks for putting up with me when I'm apprehensive before I work nights, and when I ruminate afterwards about clinical signs and symptoms I might have missed. To my children, Kaille and Sasha, your giggles remind me that there's much more to life than the ER and medical journalism, no matter how captivating and fulfilling both are.

INTRODUCTION

Some people choose to work nights. Sometimes, the night chooses people. That's what I think happened to me. On a spring night back in 1982, two years before I joined the staff at Mount Sinai Hospital, I was moonlighting in the ER of a community hospital in the heart of one of Toronto's ethnic neighbourhoods. A maintenance worker at the hospital, a man in his early sixties, checked into the ER, complaining of pain in his belly and nausea.

"I think maybe I got some food poisoning," he told one of the ER nurses. She mentioned it to me, and for some reason my radar went on alert. Though I was inexperienced back then, one thing I knew was that some patients greatly downplay their symptoms. This man was of Eastern European extraction and quite macho in a quiet way, the type who would be embarrassed to admit he was feeling too unwell to do his job. If he had spoken to a nurse about feeling a little ill, there was a good chance his true symptoms were far more serious.

When I examined him, he said he had eaten a chicken salad sandwich and all he really needed to do was throw it up. "Help me puke it, okay? Then I get back to work," he said. He gave me a quick smile that suggested there was no need to fuss over him. My gut, however, said otherwise. I don't know why, but a little voice—I tend to have this inner dialogue with myself when I assess patients—said this man was in imminent danger.

I took his history and learned he had high blood pressure, diabetes and high cholesterol. Then I ran my hand over his belly. When doctors press the abdomen for tenderness, we're checking to see if you have signs of a surgical condition like appendicitis. That night, for reasons that escape me still, I put my right hand on the maintenance worker's abdomen and slid it toward his belly button, *expecting* to feel something deadly. And that is exactly what I found.

Inside his abdomen, right in the middle, was a pulsating bulge; it felt like a tire that was about to explode, and it measured nine centimetres across. He had an aneurysm in the aorta, the major blood vessel that comes off the left ventricle of the heart and feeds the vital organs. I reckoned the aneurysm was at the level of his navel, at or below the renal arteries that feed the kidneys. At more than three centimetres in diameter, an abdominal aorta is enlarged. At five centimetres you operate. At nine you panic. If it had burst at home or while he was working he would have bled to death.

I needed to get a surgeon to operate on the man immediately and went to the nearest phone to see who was on call. As I did I passed by the nurse who had first told me to check the man out. "Food poisoning, right?" she said. I tried to resist a gloating expression. "Try abdominal aortic aneurysm," I said. "Oh my God!" she replied.

It was just after five in the morning. Could I get the on-call surgeon to come to the ER right away? I was still new to the job and had no sense of how he would respond. I was about ten seconds into my description of the problem when he said, "Wait. Let me guess. You think the patient has an aortic aneurysm." I was dumbfounded that he had guessed so quickly—and grateful that he was in sync with me. "We better get a vascular surgeon there right away."

He himself roused the vascular surgeon at home. By 6:15 the surgeon had arrived and was ready to get into action. I'll never forget waiting to see if I'd wasted my surgical colleague's time while they examined the man's belly. After they were finished, one of them turned to me and winked his approval. That's about as high praise as you get in emergency medicine.

When the surgical team was ready to operate on the man, they asked if I'd like to scrub in, meaning assist in the procedure. It was a sign of respect, an acknowledgement that I had acted professionally in a way they appreciated. I eagerly accepted the invitation.

The surgeons filled me in on what had happened before I arrived in the operating room. The minute they opened the man up the aneurysm exploded. This often happens when the aorta is weak and the air pressure inside the belly cavity equalizes with that of the operating room. Fortunately, the team was expecting it; coolly, the vascular surgeon clamped the aneurysm and spent the next two hours sewing in a graft made of Dacron. After surgery, the patient was transferred to the ICU. He went home healthy ten days later.

As I left the ER that morning, I was exhausted, high on adrenaline and in awe. Had I agreed with the nurse's first impression of food poisoning, I would probably have advised the man to drink some clear fluids and to ease off the chicken. And I'd have sent him home to a certain death. Something both mysterious and wonderful had stopped me.

This story captures many of the critical challenges I've faced working nights in the ER. Like the cop, the paramedic or the firefighter, I have the job of providing an essential service while you sleep. When you've worked at emergency medicine as long as I have, you learn to assume that people don't leave a nice, warm bed at night to come to the ER unless they have, or think they have, a life-threatening problem. It's my job to figure out what that is. Unlike your family doctor, who has known you for years, you and I have just met. I have to learn to size you up pretty quickly.

Sometimes, as was the case with the maintenance man, I may have to ignore an incorrect first impression formed by a nurse or a paramedic. To make the right diagnosis, I may have to dismiss the smell of alcohol on a patient's breath or the stench of vomit on his pyjamas. Often, I have to look past a homeless person's dishevelled appearance, or the whininess of an anxious patient's voice.

Every patient is suffering some degree of pain, either real or imagined, and ER physicians encounter both. Every patient is afraid of something: death or a life-changing disease or an inconvenient period of recuperation from a minor ailment. When they first come in their fear is usually of the unknown. "What's wrong with me, doctor?" is a typical question, even if it's not spoken out loud. But it's in their eyes; it hovers in the air as I take down their medical histories. Some ask an even tougher question: "Am I going to die?" They want answers and sometimes I have them, even if they're not the answers they want or pray to hear.

But sometimes I don't know what's wrong. Or the answers I offer are incorrect. But to survive as an ER doctor, I have to be right far, far more often than not. And I have to be right on the run, spending as little time with patients as necessary. It's not because I don't want to take longer but because I don't have that luxury: there's a waiting room full of patients. I try to work as quickly as I can on little or no sleep—a fact of life for an ER doctor.

And even when ER doctors manage to arrive at the right diagnosis, we often run into other challenges. The hospital functions with reduced staff at night. Unless a patient needs emergency surgery, the ordinarily bustling operating room is closed. So is the X-ray department. If needs be, I can obtain simple x-rays and even a CT scan of the head or a CT scan for kidney stones. However, If I want to order a CT scan of a patient's belly or chest, I have to page the radiologist on call and convince her that the scan can't wait until morning. If I feel a patient needs an emergency operation, I have to convince a sleepy surgeon to get out of bed and come to the hospital. I'd better be right, or the surgeon soon learns to doubt my pleas for help.

By sounding the alarm on the maintenance worker, I saved his life. I was twenty-six and this was my first taste of having saved a person seemingly earmarked for death. I didn't know it then, but that was the beginning of a lifelong career.

When rookies get a coveted spot on the duty roster of a hospital emergency department, they can expect to work mainly nights. In part it's a hazing ritual. I've heard many a mentor tell a resident: "I suffered through nights, and so can you." Giving nights to the young 'uns reveals another telling fact. As we get older, many of us find it hard, if not impossible, to stay alert and sharp when the sun is long gone.

When I was a newbie, back in 1982, I became the midnight man at York Central Hospital in Richmond Hill, Ontario, a bedroom community just north of Toronto. For several years, I worked ten or twelve night shifts a month, usually from 11:30 p.m. until 7:30 a.m. Back then I expected I'd pay my dues and gradually earn my way onto shifts that were more physiologically agreeable.

A funny thing happened along my journey to a decent work schedule. I realized I *love* working nights. During the daytime, I was distracted by all manner of unsolicited phone calls, which the ward secretaries were only too delighted to refer to me. Usually the calls came from doctors who wanted to send a patient to the ER. At night, calls like that almost never happen.

I also love the kinds of patients who inhabit the ER when the sun goes down. Many are anxious, some desperate, some crazy, and a few face imminent death. It's not easy to deal constantly with people in need. A family doctor encounters a wide range of cases on a daily basis, from someone with a life-threatening illness to a regular, friendly patient who just needs a prescription renewed. There's an ebb and flow of crisis and calm in the family doctor's office. Not so in the ER. The only people we encounter who don't have a genuine medical emergency have something else wrong with them, usually a mental issue or an addiction problem, and they can be as difficult to treat, if not more so, than those with a broken arm or a gnawing pain in their stomach.

There's another reason why I love working nights. It gives me plenty of time to nurture my career in medical journalism. Since the early 1980s, I've been both an ER physician at Mount Sinai Hospital in downtown Toronto and a medical journalist. During my dual career, I've made it my mission to demystify the world of medicine. My work for CBC Radio led to a career on CBC Television, first as a correspondent on *The Health Show,* a half-hour current affairs TV series, and later on *The National* as its health reporter.

Along the way, I began to take note of the things doctors, nurses and other health professionals would say to each other in hospital corridors and medical lounges—beyond the earshot of patients and members of the public. I was determined to reveal the culture of medicine and what doctors, nurses and other health professionals think and feel about patients and the system. I discovered that an important purpose of my professional life was not just to help people who needed medical care. I also wanted to treat the medical system itself, to expose the way it really is, with all its strengths, weaknesses and pretensions. As I once said to a colleague, "I'm on a mission to take the hypocritical stick out of medicine's ass. To do a 'stickec-tomy,' if I can coin a word."

That goal would be ultimately realized in 2007 with the cre-ation of *White Coat, Black Art,* a CBC Radio series that reveals the inner thoughts and stories of people who work inside the health-care system. That's when I thought of turning my experiences working nights in the ER into a book.

———————

The Night Shift: Real Life in the Heart of the ER is a book about my career and about the patients I've seen while working nights at Mount Sinai Hospital's ER and elsewhere. Its aim is to show what takes place on the other side of the ER doors, both real and figura-tive, that separate the patients from the medical staff. It's also about my approach to medicine, which has been influenced by my other career as a freelance medical journalist. I have practised both these demanding careers for nearly the same length of time.

The night shift I describe in this book is a composite of my experiences with some of the most memorable patients I've seen and treated over the years during night shifts at Mount Sinai and elsewhere. The ER at Mount Sinai is often hectic, but we don't see a lot of gore and mayhem on most nights. For this reason, freelance journalist Sam Solomon and I interviewed colleagues in emergency medicine from across Canada with stories to tell. With the CBC's permission, I also used interviews conducted by me for *White Coat, Black Art* to round out the content of the book.

I'm bound by my oath as a physician to protect patient confidentiality. I'm also bound by my compulsion to tell you what really goes on in the ER. Telling meaningful stories without violating my professional obligation takes some doing. The patients I've written about in this book are based on real people. However, I have changed their names and personal identifying information so as to protect confidentiality.

I've written this book for you. If you wake up in the middle of the night with gripping chest pain or a searing kidney stone, or if you fall out of bed and break your hip, probably your first hope is that the problem will just go away. When you realize that's wishful thinking, chances are you'll go by car or ambulance to your nearest hospital emergency department.

The statistics on ER visits are astonishing. A 2007 study found that each year nearly forty out of every one hundred North Americans visit an ER for treatment. That means sooner or later most of you are going to need the services of someone like me. Many of you will wonder just what is going on behind the ER's swinging doors, and whether your trust in the medical personnel who work there is well placed. I want to take you inside the ER, as I know it, and show you how it really operates. In doing so, I hope to demystify my profession and make your encounters in the ER more understandable and easier to handle.

At times throughout the book, I describe tests that I ordered and treatments that I either prescribed or administered. This book has been written for entertainment purposes only. It should not be taken as medical advice. For that, see your doctor.

CHAPTER ONE

A BREATH OF LIFE

FRIDAY, 9:15 P.M.

I broke into a jog on my way to the subway stop near my home in north Toronto and bolted down the steps two by two, frantic I might not make it to the hospital on time. I hate being late for a night shift. I can't bear to see the scowl on the face of a colleague who's been working his ass off all evening but can't leave until I arrive. Call me neurotic. Never the truant as a schoolchild (although I often fantasized about it), I've always fretted about being on time. I'm consistent, though. I also hate it when a colleague comes in late to relieve me.

Adding to my stress was a general anxiety that always arises just prior to a shift. Although I've been doing emergency medicine for more than twenty-five years I still get butterflies before starting work. One reason is that, despite my extensive experience, there are things I don't know and procedures I can't do as well as some of my colleagues. Few doctors will admit this, but I'm not afraid of telling the truth.

1

When my train pulled into the station I began to relax. The trip south to Mount Sinai Hospital wouldn't take long. Or so I thought. As we neared my final stop, the train shrieked to a halt. An announcement over the intercom said there was an emergency at another location, causing a "slight delay." My blood pressure rose. I cursed the wait. I hate not being in control. Thankfully, ten long minutes later, the train started inching toward my destination.

I bolted up the subway steps into the night air. I wanted to rush into the hospital, but I made a pit stop at Tim Hortons to buy a big box of Timbits for the nurses and a large coffee for me. The coffee was to keep me awake; the Timbits were for the nurses, who would remember to let me know if and when my patients were getting sicker and especially if they were about to have a cardiac arrest.

I rushed past the security desk at the Murray Street entrance to Mount Sinai, and down the steps and along a corridor to the emergency physicians' office. I changed into greens and grabbed my stethoscope. I popped a couple of modafinil pills (a medication used by many shift workers to help them stay awake) and downed them with coffee. When you're a fifty-something ER doc, you need every edge to stay awake and sharp.

I uttered the silent prayer to my patients I'd been saying since the first day I started practising emergency medicine: "Please don't come too late, and for goodness' sake, don't come too early." Timing is everything in medicine. If you come too late, I can't save you. And if you come too early, I probably won't recognize what's wrong with you because the symptoms will be too subtle.

Then, just before I started my shift, I murmured the silent prayer that I dared not say aloud: "Please don't let me screw up."

———————

On my way into the ER, I stepped into the waiting room to see how busy it was. It's a small room—thirty-seven chairs crammed into an area eleven by twelve feet. Patients, along with family and friends, occupied three-quarters of the chairs. A television set mounted in a corner of the waiting room near the outside entrance faced in toward the nurses. The seat arrangement meant that half the patients and visitors couldn't see it unless they craned their necks.

I stood just outside the swinging double doors that separated the waiting room from the ER. To my right, a nurse at the triage desk was taking a patient's blood pressure. A lineup of patients waited to register. Directly in front of me, two ambulance stretchers flanked by a crew of paramedics each bore a patient. Four more patients on ambulance stretchers formed a line that snaked along an adjoining hallway. It was going to be a very busy night.

10:00 P.M.

"Doctor Goldman, go to Resus, stat," the voice of a ward secretary blared on the intercom.

A seventy-two-year-old woman I'll call Sophia was having an epileptic seizure. Her arms and legs were jerking rhythmically and a trace of white froth had formed in her mouth. Her eyes were open and glassy and staring straight ahead. When a nurse called out to her, she didn't answer.

"She's got lung cancer and she's receiving chemo," one of the two paramedics who brought her in told me.

"Does she have a history of seizures?"

"Not that we know of," he answered as the two men transferred her from their stretcher to one of ours.

"How long has she been seizuring?"

"About two minutes," he said.

An epileptic seizure is a transient event caused by excessive or synchronous activity of the brain. Epilepsy generally means you're born with the tendency to have seizures. Other causes include scarring in the brain associated with oxygen deprivation around birth, a history of meningitis or a stroke. Another common cause is a brain tumour. Sophia's lung cancer made me fear that the disease had spread to her brain, an ominous, life-threatening development. But theorizing as to the cause would have to wait. I had to stop the seizure now. The longer it went on, the greater the risk of brain damage from lack of oxygen.

"Give her ten milligrams of diazepam," I ordered.

A nurse drew up the sedative—one of the fastest-acting drugs we have at our disposal to stop a seizure—in a syringe and injected it. Within a minute, the seizure stopped. My patient started to rouse herself. Sophia's son walked in just as the seizure ended.

"I'm Dr. Goldman, and I've been looking after your mother. Does she have a history of seizures?"

"No," he said. "Only the cancer."

I explained that the cancer had likely spread to his mother's brain. For now, we'd stopped the seizure with diazepam. I ordered an intravenous drip of a second drug, called phenytoin, to help prevent the seizures from coming back. I told him we'd keep an eye on Sophia in the resuscitation room.

"Let's get a CT scan of the head," I said to the nurse, hoping silently that there wouldn't be any cancer in the brain.

This was not the nice, easy start to my shift that I had been hoping for.

———————

As an ER physician, my first duty is to my patients. If you have a cut, a sprain or a broken bone, it's my job to patch you up and send you on your way. If you have a life-threatening illness, it's my job to keep you alive until I or someone else figures out what's wrong with you. If you want to kill yourself, it's my job to try and stop you.

My second duty is to the system. Crudely put, my job is to "move the meat." That means you. Pushing roughly 47,000 patients a year through the ER takes determination, efficiency, guile and some luck. Mount Sinai Hospital has 472 beds that are more than 90 percent occupied most of the time. Finding an available bed is a constant challenge. For every patient upstairs that doctors can't discharge, there's a patient downstairs in the ER who can't be moved upstairs, and a patient in the waiting room who can't be brought in.

I can see only one patient at a time, but there's nothing to stop countless patients from coming *ensemble,* as it were, or paramedics from bringing in a half-dozen sick people on stretchers in half an hour. We call that getting "slammed," or inundated. "The bus just pulled up," a triage nurse once sighed as she scanned a lineup of incoming patients that stretched from the registration area to the ER entrance. It's one of my favourite expressions.

We're trying to practise safe and effective emergency medicine while battling the clock. In 2001, the American Academy of Emergency Medicine released a position statement that doctors should not have to see more than 2.5 patients per hour. A report by Dr. Leslie Zun, an ER doctor in Chicago, found that various guidelines have ER physicians seeing anywhere between 1.8 and five patients per hour.

When I start an average night shift, I'm at my most efficient; I can see three to five patients per hour. Helping me do this on any given night are between ten and twelve nurses (including the ones at triage), at least one resident and maybe a medical student. I love the excitement of caring for patients like Sophia. But when someone as sick as she arrives in the resuscitation room, I have to drop everything else to tend to her, so the assembly line grinds to a halt. And even if I manage to maintain a frenetic pace, I won't be able to complete my interaction with each and every patient the first time I see them. It often takes several hours or more before the tests and X-rays or CT scans come back so that I'm able to send patients home or refer them for admission to the hospital. Invariably, as the night progresses, I have to continually reassess existing patients at the same time as I see new ones. By 4:00 or 5:00 a.m., I'm only able to handle about two new patients an hour.

Another factor that slows down an ER doctor is the frequent interruptions we have to deal with. Everyone in the ER, be it a nurse, a patient, a family member or a resident, thinks they can begin chatting with us anytime, anyplace. I've had residents walk in to tell me about their patient as I'm doing a pelvic exam on mine.

ER physician Carey Chisholm, of the Indiana University School of Medicine and the Emergency Medicine and Trauma Center at Methodist Hospital in Indianapolis, studied interruptions during the course of a typical emergency shift. He found that, on average, ER physicians were interrupted fifty-two times. In twenty-one of those instances, the interruption was so extreme it forced the ER docs to stop whatever they were doing and start something else.

In aviation, it's well known that pilot interruptions result in serious and sometimes fatal mistakes, so the industry tries to keep interruptions to a minimum. Not so in the ER. You can be trying to save a life, and a nurse will ask you for a verbal order for Tylenol. When you have the nerve to say you're too busy, some give you a look suggesting you're having a temper tantrum.

Noise is also an impediment to ER work. The ER at Mount Sinai gives off a constant barrage of mechanical alarms. The alarm that patients activate at the bedside is a two-note job with a long pause. The notes are the same as the first two in the classic rock ballad "Feelings," written by Louis "Loulou" Gasté and recorded in 1975 by Morris Albert. Every time I hear that alarm, my mind immediately begins to play the song. I can't help it.

Add to that the screams of people in pain, the delusionary wails of psychotic patients, and the constant chanting of those with Alzheimer's and other forms of dementia and you have to wonder how doctors manage to pay the attention we do.

It wasn't always this way. In 1923, the hospital opened as a thirty-three-bed maternity and convalescent facility. In 1953, the new Mount Sinai Hospital opened on University Avenue, across the street from Toronto's famed Hospital for Sick Children. In 1973, the hospital moved to its present location one door north. Today, Mount Sinai is a state-of-the-art facility that teaches medical students and residents, boasts a world-ranked research institute and cares for a growing community of complex patients. I know, because we end up seeing a lot of them in the ER.

When I started working at Mount Sinai in 1984, I saw between eight and twelve patients per shift (out of the seventy or so who passed through the swinging doors each day). Those times are long gone. Population growth plus the closure of several hospitals in the immediate vicinity mean volume has gone way up. Today, Mount Sinai's Schwartz-Reisman Emergency Centre sees 120 to 130 ER patients a day—about 47,000 a year and climbing. On some days, we see more than 160 patients. On a typical Friday night, I treat about thirty to forty patients before I hand off to the physician working the day shift that begins at 7 a.m.

It's not just the volume that's changed. It's what we call the acuity—how sick patients are. There was a time when we pre-dominantly saw patients with heart attack or pneumonia or ulcers. Now, a typical Mount Sinai patient might have diabetes, high blood pressure, heart trouble, kidney failure or cancer. Advances such as angioplasty and better chemotherapy are a mixed blessing. Patients live much longer. When I began my career, ninetysome-thing patients were a novelty; now they're commonplace.

The sliding doors between the waiting room and the ER "may as well be doors into another universe," says Dr. Wayne Pezzi, author of several medical books. Pezzi practised emergency medi-cine for more than ten years in the United States. An ER, he says, is not the glamorous or endlessly exciting trauma-filled world some TV shows make it out to be, although there are moments when that description fits.

"When people think of the ER, they think of blood and guts," says Pezzi. "They should also think of feces, urine, vomit, pus from disgusting places, unmentionable pelvic discharges, temper tan-trums, endless profanity, threats, assorted verbal abuse, and the occasional punch now and then. In fact, much of what [ER doctors] do, and must put up with, is the antithesis of glamour. It can be downright disgusting, such as when an ER doctor is disimpacting a patient [my translation: removing hard stool from the rectum]."

Unlike on TV, there's no endless stream of swinging doors being madly flung open to let a gurney through, a team of medical profes-sionals running alongside doing everything possible to save the life of a patient facing impending death. That's especially true at Mount Sinai, which does not handle gunshot or car accident victims except in rare circumstances. These cases are typically directed to other hospitals in the city specializing in those kinds of trauma.

That doesn't mean the cases at Mount Sinai are not dramatic in their own way. We treat everything from cardiac arrest to unknown rashes. A few patients are at risk of dying, but most are not. All consider their problem serious to some extent, otherwise they wouldn't have come to the hospital, where they sometimes face long and tedious hours in the waiting room.

I became an emergency physician almost by accident. In medical school, I developed an interest in neurology, the specialty that deals with strokes and other disorders of the brain. I was so taken with the field that, in my fourth year, I made what I now regard as an impulsive decision to become a child neurologist. I was accepted for an internship at the Hospital for Sick Children in Toronto. In 1979, my final year of medical school, I did a two-month rotation in neurology at Johns Hopkins Hospital in Baltimore. At the time, Johns Hopkins had a world-famous residency program in neurology. The purpose of my stint there was to catch the eye of potential mentors.

During the rotation, I started to doubt my career choice. It didn't help that I was lonely and homesick. On a critical day of my rotation, when I was scheduled to present a talk, I slept in and missed my chance to impress my higher-ups.

I returned to Toronto in crisis. It took me years to realize that a guardian angel had saved me that morning. Neurology, I now know, would have been a dead-end choice for me. Oh, I could have and would have done it well. But something creative was stirring inside my soul that would not become clear for a few years. Sleeping in saved me from years of professional and personal regret.

Still, I had applied for and been accepted as a first-year resident at the Hospital for Sick Children, in what would have been my first year of training toward becoming a child neurologist. I couldn't back out. I completed the year and transferred to what was then known as Sunnybrook Health Sciences Centre, where I did a residency year in internal medicine.

By then, I knew that I wanted to write. I had attempted to write a novel, but was unable to finish it. In July 1981, I wrote an article that was published in the science section of the *Globe and Mail*. That one success convinced me I wanted to explore my interest in writing. That's when a career in emergency medicine began to beckon. I knew fellow residents who earned extra money moonlighting in local ERs. I decided to give it a try, and soon found that emergency medicine was stimulating and intellectually satisfying. Best of all, it was part-time work that left me plenty of time to write and to work in broadcasting.

———————

Not long after I began my career as an emergency room doctor on July 1, 1982, I took part in my first cardiac arrest as a staff emergentologist. I was working night shifts at Northwestern General Hospital, located in a working-class part of Toronto.

As often happens in a workplace that deals with constant stress, such as law enforcement, journalism and medicine, seasoned staff watch (and test) the rookies to see if they can handle themselves under pressure and to determine whether they have a sense of humour. Veteran nurses and paramedics tend to be the toughest adjudicators of young doctors. They've had to deal with too many self-important recent graduates who didn't respect the vast knowledge and experience of existing staff.

One evening a male patient was brought in following a heart attack. He had been without a heart rhythm for at least ten minutes, perhaps longer. Although everyone knew he was dead, the cardiac arrest team had to try to resuscitate him nevertheless, just in case a miracle occurred. During my residency I had taken the advanced cardiac life support course, and this was an opportunity to put theory into practice. As leader of the arrest team, my role that night was to figure out why my patient's heart had stopped and how to put things right, if possible. Adhesive electrodes attached to the patient's chest told me he was in asystole: no heart rhythm and little chance of bringing him back to life.

In desperation, I charged the defibrillator and prepared to give my patient an electrical jolt of 300 joules to the heart. I put gel on the defibrillator pads and pressed them against the patient's chest, one on the right side of the breastbone and the other over the patient's left nipple. I yelled "clear," the signal for everyone in contact with the patient's stretcher to step away so they don't get an electrical shock. Following that cautionary check, I pressed the button on the defibrillator and was greeted with a brief puff of smoke and the acrid smell of singed flesh. Inadvertently, I had allowed one of the electrodes on a paddle to just catch the edge of an electrocardiograph lead, which was applied to the chest on a strip of adhesive paper. To my horror, the paper had briefly ignited.

A grizzled nurse, who looked as if she had smoked a pack or two of cigarettes a day during her decades on the job, peered at me over her bifocals and shook her head ever so slightly. "Well, if he wasn't dead before, he is now," she said, which broke everyone up. I laughed along, but I felt mortified. It was a humbling experience, and one that I'm glad took place early in my career.

Ours is a profession where mistakes can kill—not in this case, I'm happy to say; there was nothing we could have done to save this unfortunate man—and that enormous responsibility is not easy to deal with. Some doctors find it hard to admit they are human and capable of error. Some find it equally difficult to see the parts of the system that don't work well or that need improvement. If they did admit these shortfalls, they might have to question aspects of their job they'd prefer not to acknowledge or examine.

The dark-humoured nurse took me down a peg or two that day. I don't know if I needed that initiation, as I've always been harder on myself than anyone else could ever be. But it didn't hurt to go through it. It has remained a vivid memory of my potential to make a significant mistake and of the need to react with humanity—in this case, with humour and humility—when I cause something to go wrong.

I couldn't really enjoy the nurse's humour because I was terrified of freezing in a life-or-death situation, such as when you have to intubate a patient—pass a breathing tube down the patient's airway. We do this when a person's lungs are so damaged or filled with fluid that she can't breathe in enough oxygen to survive without a ventilator. We also do it when a patient's level of consciousness is so depressed by anything from a head injury to alcohol or drugs that he can't keep food or vomit from flowing up the esophagus and pouring into the lungs, a condition called aspiration. An aspirating patient can suffer a respiratory arrest right then and there, or she can die several days later of aspiration pneumonia and shock.

When I was a clinical clerk at Sunnybrook Health Sciences Centre in 1979, I had a two-week rotation in anaesthesia. That meant I had fourteen days to learn how to intubate a patient—to shove an endotracheal tube down past the vocal cords and into the trachea or windpipe. What could be simpler?

You stand behind the patient's head with the person lying face up on a stretcher and you insert an instrument called a laryngoscope into the patient's mouth. A laryngoscope is basically a six-inch handle with a retractable blade that's curved into the shape of a tongue. Without this instrument, you can't see the vocal cords; without seeing them, there's nothing to stop you from inserting the endotracheal tube into the patient's esophagus. If you do that, you'll kill the patient.

To intubate a patient, you're supposed to insert the blade over the tongue and use a groove or bracket at the side of the blade to push the tongue out of the way. If you can do that, you're supposed to inch the blade down the patient's throat or pharynx until you see the epiglottis, a big flap of skin located at the root of the tongue. The epiglottis keeps food headed toward your stomach from going down the trachea and into the lungs. If you're successful at reaching the epiglottis, you're supposed to insert the tip of the curved laryngoscope blade into a space between the root of the tongue and the epiglottis called the vallecula. If you're able to do this, you use the handle of the laryngoscope to lift the epiglottis up and out of the way (sometimes you have to lift up the patient's head). And presto, you finally see the vocal cords—the destination for the endotracheal tube.

Sounds fairly easy, no? Not so fast. If the tongue is big and floppy, it often gets in the way. Even if you can get the tongue out of the way, the epiglottis might hide the vocal cords. If the tip of the laryngoscope blade isn't quite in the vallecula, you can try lifting the epiglottis out of the way all day long and the vocal cords won't pop into view. No cords means blind intubation. As I mentioned, a blindly inserted endotracheal tube often goes into the esophagus.

You learn by practising first on a mannequin. Then you practise under supervision in the operating room on live human beings. That's when you discover that almost everyone is shaped differently from the mannequin. You discover that obese people, especially the ones with fat necks, are a lot more difficult to intubate. You find out that older people with arthritis are also tough because you can't move their necks into a good position.

Unfortunately, during my two-week rotation in anaesthesia back in med school, my "mentor" was a burned-out man in late middle age. The first morning of my rotation he left me alone with a patient during an operation well underway. "I'm going now to prepare my lunch," he said. He held up a couple of half-filled syringes. "If the patient's blood pressure goes up, give him an inch of this. If he bucks, give him an inch of that." He then walked out of the operating room before I could ask a question.

This was the guy who was supposed to teach me how to intubate. When I had trouble getting big fat tongues out of the way, he laughed. When I had trouble locating the vocal cords, he said I lacked the brute strength to lift the head out of the way. This was years before I saw all kinds of petite women do it. How was I to know that proper positioning, not brute strength, was the secret of successful intubation?

No matter how many times I tried, I couldn't intubate. I was starting to get frustrated. So was my so-called mentor. On the last day of my rotation, he was determined that I master the technique.

He anaesthetized and paralyzed the patient and handed me the laryngoscope blade. I worked hard to get the tongue out of the way until I was finally able to get the blade past the tongue. For the first time, I could see the epiglottis. But I couldn't see the vocal cords. I struggled for what seemed like another minute. The patient started to show signs of respiratory distress and was moments away from suffering cardiac arrest. The anaesthetist took the laryngoscope away from me, pulled it out, and began to ventilate the patient manually with an Ambu bag, a handheld device used to ventilate a patient until you can get a ventilator set up. The patient stabilized. I breathed deeply.

The anaesthetist handed the laryngoscope back to me and insisted I try again. This was 1979, and students didn't refuse their mentors' requests. I complied. He kept needling me to try harder to lift the head. Still, I couldn't see the vocal cords. This went on for what seemed like another two minutes—pushing the patient peril-ously close to a cardiac arrest.

When it was past clear that it was my lesson or the patient's life, the anaesthetist bowed to the inevitable. In a panic, he shoved me aside and put the tube in himself.

I was traumatized by the experience for years afterward. True, my teacher, a seasoned anaesthetist, was there to take over. So tech-nically, the patient's life wasn't in danger. But to an impressionable mind, it felt like that. And it seemed to me that the anaesthetist was more concerned about a "teachable moment."

I covered up that sense of failure through much of my early and middle career as an emergency physician. From 1984 until 2003, I had a successful career as an ER physician at Mount Sinai while rarely having to intubate a patient. Back then, you didn't have to. The patients we saw seldom needed it. In those rare instances when intubation was necessary, we enlisted the on-call anaesthetist to do it for us.

My inability to intubate made me feel inadequate as an ER doc. I'm a general practitioner (GP) emergency physician. I got my general licence back in 1982. Back then, you could start a career as an emerg doc simply by working in the ER. Oh, I passed all kinds of examinations in the years ahead. In 1986, I got my Certificate of Special Competence in Emergency Medicine from the College of Family Physicians of Canada. In 1992 I passed the written and oral examinations set by the American Board of Emergency Medi-cine. Those successes were powerful evidence that I belonged in the club of ER docs.

But I have never done a residency in emergency medicine. As a result, I missed years of training in everything from orthopedics to plastic surgery to intensive care, and, not surprisingly, anaesthesia. My much younger colleagues had learned five different techniques of difficult intubations. They were smart, better educated and a lot slicker at handling a laryngoscope than I was. By 2002, I found myself beginning each shift with a silent prayer that no patient arrive in need of emergency intubation.

Then came the outbreak that changed everything. On November 16, 2002, the first known case of atypical pneumonia occurred in Foshan City, in Guandong Province in China. By February 2003, health officials from Guandong Province reported a total of 305 cases and five deaths from acute respiratory disease. On February 21, 2003, a sixty-four-year-old medical doctor from Zhongshan University in Guandong Province arrived in Hong Kong for a wedding. He checked into the ninth floor of the Metropole Hotel. A day later, the doctor was admitted to the intensive care unit at the Kwong Wah Hospital with respiratory failure. By March 4, 2003, he was dead.

On February 23, 2003, a seventy-eight-year-old woman from Toronto checked out of the Metropole Hotel in Hong Kong for a return flight to Canada. On March 5, the woman died at Toronto's Scarborough Grace Hospital. Her forty-four-year-old son would be the next Canadian to die. Officials from the World Health Organization labelled the new disease severe acute respiratory syndrome or SARS. It would be some time before scientists at the Michael Smith Genome Sciences Centre in Vancouver, British Columbia, and the National Microbiology Laboratory in Winnipeg, Manitoba, identified the virus that caused the disease. About 8,500 persons worldwide were diagnosed with probable SARS during the epidemic, and there were over 900 deaths. In Canada, there was a total of 438 probable cases and forty-four deaths. There weren't that many cases, but the death rate was staggering. If you got this infection, you were in for the fight of your life.

I was working a set of nights when Dr. Allison McGeer, who became one of Canada's leading authorities on SARS, examined the first cluster of seriously ill patients who had been transferred from Scarborough Grace Hospital. "I don't know what we're dealing with," said McGeer. At the time, doctors hadn't yet identified the virus. I remember asking her if it could be a pandemic strain of influenza.

"Could be," she said.

Turns out it wasn't. SARS wasn't a virus that spread readily from person to person. You had to have prolonged exposure to the cough secretions of an infected patient to be at risk of getting the disease. Health-care workers were especially vulnerable. More than one hundred in Canada contracted SARS. That number included at least one anaesthetist at Mount Sinai and at least one respiratory therapist. Suddenly, during the spring and summer of 2003, it became much more common for ER staff like me to intubate our patients, many of whom arrived with fever and respiratory distress and were suspected of having SARS.

Fortunately, this time I had some great teachers. I have no idea what they thought of me, a doctor in his late forties asking to be taught how to intubate. I approached Dr. Ivor Fleming, an anaesthetist who at the time took care of the duty roster. He paired me up with anaesthetists who patiently taught me the proper technique.

This time, I got it. Slowly but surely, with the help of anaesthetists like Fleming, Gord Urbach and Gordon Fox, I began to feel comfortable with a laryngoscope blade in my hand. More importantly, they taught me newer rescue techniques that can keep a patient alive and well oxygenated until help arrives.

I'll never forget the first time I did a crash intubation in the ER after my period of retraining. The patient was a thirty-year-old who had become a quadriplegic years earlier in a car accident. He was prone to severe pneumonia, and had required intubation and an admission to the intensive care unit mere months earlier.

One look at the guy told me he was minutes away from having

a respiratory arrest. His face was a dusky blue colour, the telltale sign of cyanosis. His breathing was laboured and shallow. He was disoriented from lack of oxygen. I knew this was the moment to intubate him myself. I called for a respiratory therapist to assist me. I prepared to use a technique called rapid sequence intubation, or RSI. Basically, you give the patient oxygen, something to sedate him, something to anaesthetize him and something to paralyze him. All in a five-minute span. Then you intubate.

My heart was pounding as I gave the nurses their orders.

The moment I administered succinylcholine, the paralyzing drug, I experienced that sick, giddy feeling I imagine skydivers get as they stand in the open door of an airplane, waiting to jump with a parachute. Like all skydivers, I always have a backup chute—a sure-fire technique I can use, in case I can't intubate, that can keep the patient alive long enough to try a second time, or to call an anaesthetist to take over. But until the paralyzing drug wore off, his life was in my hands.

I held my breath as I waited for my patient to twitch, a muscular reaction called fasciculation that happens the moment before the patient is completely paralyzed. Thirty seconds later, his muscles twitched. I inserted the laryngoscope blade over his tongue. I was amazed at how much more easily it went in with the patient paralyzed. I found the epiglottis right away. Unlike all the other times that I had trouble with the vallecula, this time the tip of the laryngoscope blade made purchase with it.

I lifted the handle of the laryngoscope, and I was treated to the most perfect view of the vocal cords I have seen before or since. I slipped the endotracheal tube in with ease, as if I'd been doing it my entire career.

Since then, I've turned my trouble intubating into an advantage. Like the mediocre athlete who becomes a great coach, I've become a pretty good teacher of airway management. I have a lot to offer students and residents because I had to deconstruct the technique many times over until I could get it right.

And I'm a safer ER doc because, when I intubate, I'm always aware of just how quickly things can go wrong.

———————————

Another incident early in my career has also shaped my approach to working in the ER. A man who had been admitted to another hospital with mental health problems had left, or "eloped" as we say, of his own accord. A short while later he entered the subway system and jumped in front of a train, dying instantly. Paramedics at the hospital where I worked at the time brought his body back to the hospital because he had to be officially pronounced dead.

They took him into a side room and placed him on a bed with a sheet covering all but his head. I had not seen a lot of corpses at this point, and it was always a solemn moment for me to gaze at a lifeless being. His eyes were closed as if he were asleep, finally at peace from the demons that had infected his mind. When I pulled the sheet back, however, I was instantly repelled. I was unaware that the train had decapitated him. As a joke, the paramedic crew had flipped his torso over, so his head was facing up but the rest of his body was turned the opposite way. I didn't find it funny at all and I almost threw up.

What the paramedic crew did that night was an indignity. I have a black sense of humour and readily enjoy the relief provided by a biting comment such as the one the nurse aimed at me during the failed defibrillation. This, however, was way over the line. To be fair, the incident happened more than two decades ago. The paramedics I know and work with today are humble and sensitive, and the sense of professionalism among them is immense. I haven't heard of a prank like that in recent years, and I would be very surprised to hear of it happening today. It's true that people in the medical profession can become inured to death and illness and pain because we witness so much of them. But I don't think we should become so callous that we find the suicide of a troubled person the inspiration for a gag. In doing so, we risk losing touch with our feelings and our connection to what our patients and their loved ones are going through when we encounter them in the ER. I never want that to happen to me. That horrifying image, which I can still see, serves as a constant reminder to treat everyone I come in contact with as a doctor the same way I would want my family and friends to be treated.

10:45 P.M.

I checked on Sophia in the resuscitation room, where she was slowly waking up from her seizure. The CT scan of her head confirmed my worst fears. The lung cancer had deposited its deadly spores in her brain. She would need radiation to try and shrink the tumours. The news was as good as a death sentence.

But there was more. A chest X-ray showed a large accumulation of fluid on the left side of the chest, yet another deadly consequence of the cancer. The fluid was not inside the lung itself. Rather, it was occupying what was normally a very small area called the pleural space, located between the inside of the chest wall and the lung. I estimated there were at least two litres of cancerous liquid in the chest cavity. There was no way she could go home. I asked a resident to admit her.

I moved on to my next patient, not knowing that, just a few hours later, I would have to save Sophia's life again.

CHAPTER TWO

MATTERS OF THE HEART AND WOMB

11:00 P.M.

The next case was most unusual, one I had never encountered before in my career and likely never will again. It began with a woman's agonizing scream, which reverberated through the department with a Doppler effect, quieting down then ramping up, as if the woman was being moved from one room to another.

It's not out of the ordinary to hear loud screaming in the ER. Often it's an agitated psychiatric patient or someone in excruciating pain who has yet to receive medication. The screaming stopped, so I decided to begin my night by looking in on another patient. As I was about to do so the howling erupted again. Now I'm a pain doctor, which means I'm absolutely committed to relieving pain whenever and however I can. I headed to the source of the high-pitched yowls to see what I could do to alleviate the woman's obvious discomfort.

Leticia was about thirty and whip-thin. She was lying on her back, one hand desperately clutching that of an older woman, who turned out to be her mother. The triage nurse had noted that Leticia had been experiencing severe abdominal pain for several hours that night, which is why she had come to the ER.

Leticia was quiet as I began to do what we call an abdominal pain workup—detailing as much information related to her situation as I could obtain from her.

"Have you been vomiting? Had nausea? Fever? Diarrhea? Trouble peeing?" I asked. She said no to all.

When Leticia suddenly arched her back and emitted another impressive scream I thought she might have a kidney stone. I wanted to prescribe a painkiller but needed a clearer sense of her problem before I could make a decision on what to administer. She calmed down within a few moments, which allowed me to put my hand on her abdomen. Although she was scrawny I could feel a slight protuberance, but nothing dramatic. It was rigid, which now suggested peritonitis, an inflammation of the membrane that lines part of the abdominal cavity, often caused by an infection and treatable with antibiotics. As I was mulling over this possibility she convulsed once again, shrieking in agony for a few moments before collapsing back on the bed.

It's startling what can go through your mind at times. As I began to deduce what was really happening with Leticia, I thought about urban myths, those fantastical tales of gruesome events or incredible coincidences that turn out to be false. In medicine, one such legend is about a medical student about to dissect his first cadaver. He pulls back the sheet and to his horror sees that it's someone he knows; often it's his kindergarten teacher, for some bizarre reason. Another is about a woman in her third trimester (at least twenty-four weeks after conception) or beyond who has no idea she is pregnant. It's a great story but not one any doctor would really swallow. No woman, it was thought, could be that far advanced in pregnancy without knowing what was happening to her body. That was my understanding, too—until I treated Leticia.

We rarely deliver babies in the ER at Mount Sinai. On the odd occasion we've had to race out to a taxicab or car pulled up in front of the ER to assist a mother just as she's gone into the final stages of labour. But most times when a woman about to give birth shows up we send her immediately to the delivery ward. If she's less than twenty weeks pregnant, however, we're supposed to handle her in the ER, since she needs medical treatment, not obstetrical. If we bounce her up to the delivery suite, they send her back to us along with an angry note reminding us of the proper procedure.

Before saying anything to Leticia about my suspicions I took out my stethoscope and checked for a fetal heartbeat. I found one drumming away at 150 beats per minute. I moved the stethoscope a few centimetres and found another heart rate, this one at eighty beats (a normal adult heart rate is sixty to one hundred).

I looked at Leticia and her mother and could tell they had no idea about her condition. "I think I know what's causing your pain," I said. I had to suppress a devilish desire to smile. They both looked at me for the answer. I paused a moment and then addressed Leticia.

"You're pregnant," I said softly. You're in pain because you're in labour."

It would be an understatement to say they were shocked. I'll never forget the expression on Leticia's face. It was like from those horror films where Freddy Kruger or some other attacker is chasing the victim and she finally realizes she's not going to get away. She turns to face him knowing this is the end.

"No," she gasped. "It's not possible."

I turned up the stethoscope, put it in her ears, and guided it over the two heartbeats. When it came to the baby's more rapid beat I asked her: "What do you think that is?" Leticia stared open-mouthed at her mother, who was as much in shock as her daughter. A discovered pregnancy usually elicits happiness. Not this time.

As I arranged for Leticia to be transferred to the delivery ward, I asked whether she had any support beyond her mother, who seemed kind and concerned but had a tired demeanour, as if she had a lot to deal with in life. Although I could have been wrong, my sense was that they were not well off financially, and this surprise baby was not going to improve their lot. My question was also an indirect way of trying to determine if the baby's father was involved in Leticia's life. Her chart said she was married, but that didn't mean she and her husband were together.

"My husband is working out of the province," she said. "He won't be back for a few more months." Leticia was in active labour, and this was not the time to probe any further into her personal life, especially as to whether the absent husband was the child's father. I told the two women about the various social services available to them and wished them well. I found out a short time later that she had delivered a baby girl who was healthy despite being quite premature. A sweet little "myth," I said to myself.

When I talked about the case to the resident on duty later that night, I told her about an *Annals of Emergency Medicine* study conducted some fifteen years earlier. It revealed that seven out of every hundred women who attended the ER and were found to have a positive pregnancy test had no idea they had conceived. "The teaching point," I noted, "is that we should never assume that a woman of child-bearing potential isn't pregnant. Never. They are all potentially pregnant until proven otherwise. This understanding changes everything. Appendicitis suddenly becomes an ectopic pregnancy and you can't afford to be wrong about that." (An ectopic pregnancy is a dangerous situation in which the fertilized egg implants itself somewhere other than in the uterus, usually in the fallopian tubes.)

11:19 P.M.

Mario, an eighty-four-year-old gentleman, was my next intriguing patient. He had come in a few hours earlier accompanied by his son and daughter-in-law, who seemed annoyed with Mario's seemingly lackadaisical attitude toward his situation. My resident, who was top notch, told me Mario had been complaining of weakness in his left arm and leg since the night before. He was also having trouble standing on his own. Earlier that day he had been swimming, the first time he'd felt strong enough to exercise since he had experienced a fall some three weeks before. During the swim, however, he had a momentary spell of weakness, which led to his children's insistence that he come in for a checkup.

Mario's symptoms suggested a stroke, especially considering his age. But he did not mention experiencing a facial droop—a sagging on one side of the face usually due to muscle paralysis—or slurred speech, both of which should have accompanied a stroke. Nor was he complaining of a headache or vomiting. But there was no question his left side was weaker, a point made clear when a nurse grabbed the fingers on each of his hands. The left did not have the same strength as the right.

"I'm fine," he told me, proudly mentioning that he played golf several times a week and power walked as much as he could. "I'm old. That's my only problem. I shouldn't be wasting your time when you could be helping people who are really sick." I'd heard this line many times before, especially from elderly patients like Mario who, I learned, had not spent much time in hospital. Sometimes I think that people who are disinclined to seek medical help are more likely to avoid illness than those who come running to a doctor or hospital at any hint of a problem. Can we will sickness away? I doubt many of my colleagues would be comfortable suggesting that could be the case. We certainly don't want genuinely ill people trying to cure themselves just by chanting a mantra or thinking positively, although those actions can't hurt. I liked Mario's spunk, but I felt certain something was indeed wrong with him medically.

"I think you may have had a stroke, sir," I told him, a diagnosis my resident shared. "Something we call a transient ischemic attack, or a mini-stroke. The blood supply to your brain was likely blocked for a short while, and then it was restored. The good news is that it wasn't a major stroke. The not-so-good news is that it's often a harbinger of a future stroke, unless we take measures to reduce that happening."

One thing most laypeople don't know about strokes is that there's not much you can do about them once they've happened unless you see the patient within a few hours of the event. After about twelve to twenty-four hours, our only real treatment is to work on preventing a reoccurrence. If Mario had indeed experienced a stroke, it might have happened recently enough that we could administer a clot-busting drug to unblock his clogged artery, something you want to do if possible.

This is not a course of action to be taken without careful consideration. The drug has no benefit if given too late after a stroke. It also has a serious potential side effect: it can cause a cerebral hemorrhage. For cautionary reasons, we have implemented a code stroke protocol in the ER. This requires that a CT scan be taken to ensure there's no bleeding in the brain. CT stands for computerized tomography. A thin X-ray beam rotates 180 degrees around a patient's body and provides a two-dimensional image. It is about a hundred times clearer than a normal X-ray. If there is bleeding, the drug could prove fatal, a terrible outcome I knew had happened in other cases.

There was a nagging detail in Mario's history that made me wonder whether his symptoms might be caused by something else. He said he had fallen three weeks earlier. What he hadn't mentioned the first time is that he'd slipped backwards and hit the back of his head. A brief loss of consciousness was followed by complaints of light-headedness, which Mario typically downplayed. It sounded as if he might have suffered a possible concussion.

My resident impressed me with how she had probed the mechanism of Mario's accident. When an elderly patient falls, a doctor wants to know whether it's because he tripped or because he lost consciousness. If he tripped you can relax. He was probably clumsy or bumped into a piece of furniture. But if he was just walking along and suddenly blanked, then came to on the floor without knowing what happened, that's a more serious problem. It's called syncope— a fainting spell—and suggests the person has a heart rhythm disturbance, until proven otherwise. The person has to be admitted to hospital and undergo a battery of tests under the care of a cardiologist. "I just tripped," Mario insisted, although we weren't sure he was telling the truth.

Mario didn't like the sound of a CT scan, but when I explained to his son that I couldn't contemplate giving him the clot-busting drug, which he might require, until I saw the results of the scan, he convinced his father to co-operate. Thank God we insisted on following the protocol. When the resident and I looked at the scan an hour or so later we both said the same thing virtually in unison: "Holy shit!" Mario, it turned out, had incurred a subdural hematoma from the fall, an injury similar to but less lethal than the one that would kill actress Natasha Richardson after a skiing accident in March 2009. A subdural is a traumatic head injury that causes bleeding in the brain. It can have an immediate effect on the victim or it can linger, like a ticking bomb, and go off days or weeks or even months later. Mario was lucky to be alive. He needed to be seen by a neurosurgeon right away. That meant moving him to a hospital that had a neurosurgeon on duty, which was not the case at Mount Sinai.

I telephoned Toronto Western Hospital to see if they had an available bed. One of the most depressing aspects of my job is hunting for a bed for a patient who urgently needs attention. We are often told that none is available. Toronto Western employed a nurse who acted as a patient flow coordinator, or "bed czar" as we tended to call her. She was responsible for determining whether a bed was available at TWH or, if not, at another hospital. "I've been called a bed nazi," Ruth Abbott, one of the original bed czars at Toronto Western Hospital, once said with a smile.

I once had a patient who came to Mount Sinai complaining of a stiff neck and "the worst headache of my life." She needed to be in a darkened room because she had photophobia, meaning she was extremely sensitive to light. When I heard those symptoms I immediately worried that she had a subarachnoid hemorrhage—bleeding in the brain, most likely from a ruptured aneurysm. The "arachnoid" part of the term refers to the spider-web structure of the membrane that encloses the spinal cord and brain. If a ruptured aneurysm isn't fixed—it needs to be clipped or capped off with a coil or with a kind of cement—it can burst and kill or badly harm the patient.

This woman had checked into another hospital's ER a few days before. The physician who saw her had correctly ordered a CT scan, which did not reveal a subarachnoid hemorrhage. He concluded that she just had a terrible headache, prescribed some Tylenol 3s and sent her home. When the headache persisted, her instincts told her it warranted a second opinion, which brought her to us.

Studies show that CT scans pick up 95 percent of subarachnoid hemorrhages; still, they miss the remaining 5. I'm guessing the ER physician at the other hospital knew that too. I assume he did what many of us (including me) have done from time to time: he decided to take a small risk that she was in the 95 percent grouping when he sent her home.

I felt certain the woman had an aneurysm and ordered another CT scan, which found the hemorrhage. My patient was in imminent danger, as we had no way of knowing if or when the aneurysm would burst. My next step was to call the provincial office that takes down the patient's information and then tries to find a bed in a neurosurgical facility somewhere in Ontario. Often, this may involve repeating the same story to more than one neurosurgeon, only to find there isn't a bed available to take the patient. The office called me back soon after with a message that made my blood boil and freeze at the same time: "Dr. Goldman, I'm sorry but there are no available neurosurgical beds in the entire province of Ontario. We are going to continue looking, but if we don't find one she is going to Buffalo. Please make sure she and her family members have their passports with them just in case."

She indeed ended up being taken to Buffalo, about 160 kilometres away. I was later told the operation was a success and she made a complete recovery, no thanks to our overloaded and under-resourced medical system.

Mario was more fortunate. Toronto Western had a bed for him. When I went to tell the family the news, they were in the midst of a small squabble. Mario's son was pressuring him to admit that his condition since the fall had been worse than he'd let on. After a bit of prodding, Mario confessed that he hadn't been the same since the accident. It was a difficult admission for a proud man. He was taken to Toronto Western later that night, where he was operated on, and he made a full recovery.

"It's a good thing we didn't jump to conclusions," I said to the resident as we debriefed the case. "You listened to everything he said, not just to information that confirmed our suspicion of a stroke. Good work." She appreciated the praise, as we all do when we know it's been earned. Mentally I gave myself a little pat on the back too.

11:34 P.M.

Some cases touch you on a universal level—there's something about the person involved or the specifics of the circumstances that evokes an unexpected response within you—while other cases reach a personal part of you that you'd prefer to keep separate from your work. That's hard to do in the ER, and in medicine in general, because all of us have some illness or loss in our lives.

The next significant patient I saw triggered a painful memory that, due to the unfortunately common nature of her condition, arose too often for my liking.

The patient was a thirty-year-old pregnant woman who arrived complaining of vaginal bleeding and a stabbing abdominal pain. She was married with no children. We have a nomenclature in medicine for pregnant women—G refers to how many times the woman has been pregnant, P to how many times she has given birth, and M to how many times she has miscarried. Adele was G3P0M2, meaning this was her third pregnancy; the first two had not produced a child. After speaking with her I learned she had lost both previous pregnancies to first-term miscarriages.

The vaginal bleeding had begun thirty-six hours earlier, and it was often heavy. She was passing clots, although not placenta. She had severe pain on both sides of her abdomen and constant aching throughout her body. I knew the odds were high she was going through a third miscarriage. One is bad enough. Three can be emotionally devastating, bringing a sense that this will be the outcome of every pregnancy, which is not necessarily true. I knew I would have to impart the sad news, and there was no easy way to do that. We see a lot of miscarriages in the ER.

I am never detached when I deal with women or couples who come to the ER with concerns about a pregnancy. I remember too clearly the image of the gynecologist telling my wife, Tamara, and me the same bad news in a manner that seemed so detached, although it was probably just his way of managing his discomfort. I remember even more vividly all the frightening and painful moments of not knowing the outcome of a pregnancy and then knowing it only too well.

Tamara and I were married on December 21, 1996. We both wanted children, and because of our ages—Tamara was thirty-seven and I was three years older—that meant trying to get pregnant right away. Unfortunately, Tamara's first pregnancy ended in a miscarriage, and her second in a rare but dangerous condition known as partial trophoblastic disease. This is a very abnormal pregnancy caused by a weird welding of three sets of chromosomes. The problem is that this sort of tissue can turn into a potentially fatal form of cancer called choriocarcinoma. The only way to prevent that is to refrain from becoming pregnant for up to a year or longer. By the time we were given the go-ahead to try again, Tamara was forty years old.

We tried in-vitro fertilization and other forms of assisted reproduction without success. Eventually, we became parents by adopting two children from Russia. We adopted our daughter, Kaille, in 1999 and our son, Sasha, in 2002.

As I told Adele and her husband the sad news, which they had already sensed, I wanted to say to her that I knew how she felt. I wanted to turn to her husband and offer some words that might help console him. Sometimes I'm not affected by a miscarriage, but on other occasions—and I never know why—I am reminded of my own loss. I didn't share my personal story, of course. It wasn't appropriate. It would have deflected their pain and grief away from themselves and toward me. They had a right to their suffering, as Tamara and I had some ten years before.

The understandably upset couple wanted to know why she had miscarried. Frankly, we seldom if ever know the exact reason. Perhaps there was a problem with the egg or the sperm. Perhaps the fertilized egg didn't implant inside the womb properly. Many couples want to know if they did something wrong. Recently, a woman was in tears because she thought that a glass of alcohol had ended the pregnancy. I try to tell couples that babies are resilient to more than a glass of alcohol. I'm tempted to tell them I've seen many women who abuse their bodies with cocaine and crystal methamphetamine and still carry children to term. I don't say that because it would only make most of them feel worse.

Sometimes I feel pangs of envy when I see couples that learn all is well, that their pregnancy is still on track. It's not that I wish the opposite for them. It's that I wish the opposite had happened to us. Most of the time, though, I revel in telling them the good news. Recently, I had the experience of telling a woman with spotting who feared she was losing her baby that she was, in fact, carrying healthy twins—both clearly visible on an ultrasound. I shared in her happiness. My delight was genuine, and I could sense she knew it.

We're always on the run in the ER. There's always a waiting list of patients and their entourage who need our attention as soon as possible. We can't linger long with someone once we've completed our essential medical duties. But perhaps some of us hide behind that reality and use it as an excuse to remove ourselves from patients in pain and shock after they've been told bad news. Perhaps we could take an extra moment and offer a little of our humanity as well as our medical knowledge to help them cope with their suffering. I try to do that as often as I can, as do some, but not all, of my colleagues. It's my nature to act this way, but it's also my awareness of what it's like to need that comfort when it seems the world has come crashing down unfairly on your head.

CHAPTER THREE

A LONG WAIT'S JOURNEY INTO NIGHT

11:48 P.M.

As I came back to my office after seeing a patient, I passed a man snoring lightly on a gurney in the hallway. In his mid-sixties and burly, he had a bushy white beard and ruddy complexion that evoked the usual comparison to Santa Claus. I was impressed by his ability to nod off despite the endless clatter all around him and the ceaseless glare of the bright lights, which are always on in the hallway, unlike in the rooms, where they can be dimmed. He wore a baseball hat pulled down over his eyes. I didn't know how long he'd been there, but it had to be at least thirty-six hours. He had a fractured pelvis and needed to be transferred to a nearby rehabilitation facility. But there were no beds available, so for the meantime he was marooned on the gurney, sleeping on and off as best he could. I admired his disposition, which was calm and not disruptive in any way.

Another gurney was leaning against the wall directly outside my office. This one also had a man on it, and he'd been there for about seven hours. I saw from his chart that fifty-three-year-old Curtis had come in complaining of a pain on the right side of his abdomen that suggested possible appendicitis. The previous ER doctor had ordered an ultrasound, but as is often the case, it wasn't able to show the appendix. Because Curtis said he was still feeling tender on the right side, the doctor ordered a CT scan of his abdomen. Unfortunately there had been a rush for CT scans at that time and it had taken several hours for Curtis's scan to be done. The test results had not come back in.

Curtis's wife and mother had been sitting beside him in the hallway on hard chairs during his prolonged stay. He and his mother seemed resigned to the long wait, but his wife was fidgety and angry and kept getting up and pacing the halls, her displeasure obvious. I could tell she was the type of person who believed a squeaky wheel got the grease or, in this case, the results of the scan. She kept asking the nurses and me if the results had come in yet. I passed by her every time I entered my office and watched as she became increasingly annoyed. I didn't blame her. The results should have arrived several hours earlier, if not sooner.

There was no point telling her it had nothing to do with me. First of all, I had inherited her husband from the doctor on duty before I came in. Secondly, that doctor had done everything he was supposed to. I knew that my resident, who was extremely competent, was monitoring the case, as I had plenty of other patients in greater need of my attention. I didn't tell Curtis and his clan this, since I didn't want his wife bearing down on the resident.

"I have put in another request for the results," I gently told her. "They should have been back by now but I assume they're really busy." I sympathized with her and her husband. Curtis was stuck in limbo in the hallway because there was no other place to put him.

At its busiest, Mount Sinai has as many as eleven patients on stretchers in the corridors of the ER—some admitted and waiting for a bed in the hospital proper, and the rest waiting to be seen by the ER physician on duty. That's nothing compared to hospitals in other cities. In November 2009, I visited the emergency department at the Sir Mortimer B. Davis Jewish General Hospital in Montreal. Dr. Eddy Lang, a veteran of nineteen years in the ER, gave me a tour.

"In a period when flu is hitting hard, or if we have an icy day with a lot of falls and fractures, we can see a corridor [full of patients] extending all the way to the elevators on the other side and all the way out to another hallway," he told me on *White Coat, Black Art*. "All told, you can see as many as forty patients in a hallway when things are really falling apart. It's kind of like a game of chess or checkers, because our charge nurse and our physician in charge are always looking through the patient roster and saying, 'Well, who is stable enough for the hallway, and who in the hallway is now showing signs that we'd better keep a closer eye on them and bring them inside?'"

While I was there, I met Esther Levy, a woman whose mother was admitted to the corridor with heart and kidney problems. "When I brought her in three months ago, we thought she was gonna die," Levy said. "They saved her, but she was here for one week in the emergency."

Corridor patients are so endemic there that the hospital put up curtains in the hallways to create small patient cubicles.

"One of the things we realized early on is that if we're going to be holding patients in the corridor for extended periods of time, there's going to be privacy and confidentiality issues," Lang said. "Just the indignity of having to examine someone's heart and lungs with everybody walking right by and being around is just unacceptable."

Valerie Pelletier, head nurse of the emergency department, said the curtains create only an illusion of privacy: "In the main corridor, anybody can walk in like right now," she said on *White Coat, Black Art.* "We're there, and we see every patient, and we have all the family members of every other patient walking in the main corridor seeing everybody."

And yet, patients in Quebec don't seem to complain about long hospital admissions in the corridor. Esther Levy accepted that a loss of privacy was a reality caused by the volume of patients needing care. "They have a sort of curtain and they close it," she said. "What [more] do you want?"

A friend of mine had recently taken his daughter, a university student, to the ER at a Toronto hospital. She was dehydrated and complaining of stomach pains. After being brought in, she was given an IV to alleviate the immediate dehydration problem and her blood was taken and sent off for analysis. She didn't see a doctor until nine hours later. Her father griped to a triage nurse about the long delay. "I'm sorry," she said, "but that's pretty standard around here for her situation." His daughter ultimately required medication for a nasty gastrointestinal bug and was released more than ten hours after checking in. "The actual time spent treating her by the nurses and doctor was probably about half an hour," he told me. "I can't believe it took that long for her blood work to get back. Most of the time she was lying on a bed being ignored."

There's a poster in Mount Sinai's ER that says: "Waiting can be frustrating. Knowing why you may have to wait can make your visit easier." I don't know how much comfort patients and their loved ones gain if they're told the reason for a lengthy wait, but I have to believe it helps to some degree. I always make the effort to explain why delays occur. But we usually don't have the time, and sometimes we don't take the time, to explain that the main factor determining the order in which patients are treated has to do with the nature of their problem. I sense most people understand that a life-threatening condition takes priority over a broken finger. What they probably don't know is that there's a protocol governing our decisions as to who goes to the front of the treatment line.

The Canadian Triage and Acuity Scale (CTAS) categorizes ER patients on a range from 1 to 5, depending on how urgently they need care, with 1, 2 and 3 being considered urgent cases, and 1 being the highest priority.

Level 1 is "resuscitation"—patients in imminent danger of dying or who could lose a limb or suffer some other catastrophic outcome unless immediate aggressive intervention occurs.

Level 2 is "emergent"—patients who are almost but not quite in the same danger as those in level 1.

Level 3 is "urgent"—patients who have a condition that could potentially progress to a serious problem, such as vaginal bleeding and pregnancy issues, moderate head trauma, acute pain, and suicidal thoughts.

Level 4 is "semi-urgent"—less serious concerns such as headaches and back pain.

Level 5 is "non-urgent"—fairly minor complaints such as a sore throat or minor abdominal pain.

There are CTAS guidelines as to how soon a patient in each category should be seen by a doctor:

Level 1—immediately 98 percent of the time.
Level 2—within 15 minutes 95 percent of the time.
Level 3—within 30 minutes 90 percent of the time.
Level 4—within 60 minutes 85 percent of the time.
Level 5—within 120 minutes 80 percent of the time.

I would wager that ERs almost always meet the guidelines for patients in the first two categories, but CTAS 3? I'm not so sure. I think a lot of patients in that category wait hours, not the thirty minutes considered standard. As for the poor souls in the last two groupings? Many of them must wonder why they bothered coming in the first place.

The triage nurses used to attach blue cards bearing the patient's name to magnetic clips and place them on a magnetic board in order of urgency. Nowadays I find out which patient is supposed to be seen next by logging on to a computer terminal, one of many strategically located throughout the ER.

There are often fifteen to twenty patients waiting to be seen. On a typical night shift, which starts at 10:00 p.m., there could be as many as twenty or more. The number tends to decrease in the early morning hours, when fewer people show up at the ER unless they're in urgent need of help.

During the shift in question we still used the cards. My goal was to have the board cleared or down to as few cards as possible by the time I handed the shift over to the incoming doctor, between 7:00 and 8:00 a.m. That was, and still is, a source of pride to me. I don't want my replacement to inherit a backload of patients who've been waiting for hours to be seen, especially since a slew of new ones will be coming in as the new day unfolds.

"Moving the meat," as I mentioned before, is a big part of our job. If you don't move the meat, the backlog will quickly mount and the ER will become chaotic and unmanageable. Although there's no official quota, it's expected an ER doctor should be able to see three patients an hour on average. Anything less can turn a quiet shift into a disaster or a busy shift into a catastrophe. Some really fast doctors can examine five or six patients an hour, which means they're moving an awful lot of meat at an incredibly quick pace.

The hidden danger in long waiting times is that while patients are waiting to be seen the problem that brought them to the ER might get much worse. "We know that patients who are waiting prolonged periods of time before they see a physician will on occasion experience a bad outcome as a result of those delays," agreed Dr. Lang.

The nurses, of course, know which doctors are slow, average or fast. I think I am regarded as a bit faster than average.

To get a sense of just what those hourly caseload numbers mean, it's important to know that "seeing" patients—the time I spend speaking with them and/or their loved ones in their room—isn't the only time spent on their cases.

I have to first read their chart or sit down with a resident (a recent and licensed medical graduate working under our supervision), a medical student, or a nurse who might have already spoken with the patient and assessed the case. Because Mount Sinai is a teaching hospital, that interaction might involve exploring the possible causes for the patient's condition and what treatments, including medications, I might prescribe.

After dealing directly with a patient, I might have to outline the important aspects of my diagnosis to whoever came in with him. That's especially true if the patient is very elderly or a young child. If I need tests run I have to write out the orders. If the patient requires a specialist such as a neurosurgeon or a gynecologist, known in the ER as a "consult," I have to page them and speak to them. Those calls, and the responses that might come a few minutes or hours later, consume time. Depending on the case, I might have to do some research in my office—a cramped, windowless eight-by-ten-foot room that is shared by all the ER doctors; no luxury there, let me tell you. If the patient has been to Mount Sinai before, I'll look up her history on the computer. If X-rays or other tests for that patient, or someone I examined previously in my shift, have been completed and sent to me I will look them over in my office as well. That's not a definitive list but it provides an idea of all the unseen responsibilities of the ER doctor on duty.

Another factor that affects how many patients a doctor might treat in a shift is money. The Ontario government has negotiated a complicated payment structure with doctors that allows individual groups of physicians leeway as to exactly how the pay formula works. Without going into all the technical details, at Mount Sinai we've chosen a system that pays emergency doctors a fee per hour that escalates depending on the hour of day (more if you work at night, for example) plus a flat fee, which in 2009 was $35 for each patient we see.

The idea behind this formula is to give emergency physicians an incentive to treat as many patients as possible. The only downside for a doctor is that you get paid $35 whether you're dealing with a cardiac arrest or trimming a hangnail. If an ER doctor wants to pump up his income, he can do so to a certain degree by working as fast as possible. The pace I work at, however, is not motivated by money. I move as quickly as I can because I don't want to acquire a reputation as a slacker, nor do I want to hand over a large number of unfinished patients to the next shift. Whatever a doctor's motivation, it's critical that proper care of patients take overall precedence. You don't want to rush a diagnosis and risk making a mistake, nor do you want to take so much time with one patient that someone else who might urgently need your help is kept waiting.

A 2007 study by the Canadian Institute for Health Information found that patients typically waited one to four hours in Ontario's emergency rooms. The waits in small hospitals, not surprisingly, were shorter than those at large ones, with teaching hospitals in large centres such as Toronto being the slowest to treat and discharge or transfer patients to another facility. Half of the people checking into a Toronto ER were in and out within four hours. Ten percent, however, endured more than twelve hours.

A shortage of available beds contributes significantly to delays. We have only so many beds and patient rooms at the Mount Sinai ER, and if there's a crush of patients we might have to keep them in the aptly named waiting room until a bed becomes free. At the same time, for years there has been a shortage of acute care beds in other hospital departments and nursing homes, which can create a backlog at Mount Sinai and other ERs as we search for a hospital with an available bed.

Dr. Louise McNaughton-Filion, chairwoman of the Champlain Emergency Services Network in the Ottawa region, told the *Ottawa Citizen* in 2007 that "between 15 and 50 per cent of medical beds in the Champlain region are occupied by patients requiring long-term care—mainly the elderly awaiting beds in nursing homes." Dr. John Earle, chief of the emergency department at the Queensway Carleton Hospital in Ottawa, agreed. "That's what's killing us," he told the newspaper, adding that he would be able to meet the recommended benchmarks if emergency patients who need to be admitted to hospital didn't have to wait for beds.

My CBC Radio show, *White Coat, Black Art,* actually got its name as a result of the frustration some people feel when stuck waiting in an ER. After I had successfully pitched the idea for a program that would reveal how things really work in the medical profession, it was still without a name, which is a critical part of any production. One day as we were working on developing the show, my producer, Quade Hermann, kept saying, "I want to see the black art of the waiting room. Why do you wait two hours in emergency one day and fifteen minutes the next time you go in?"

I kept hearing "black art" and I began imagining these doctors walking around the ER in white coats. We have a large laminated board in our office where we write down the program's schedule and other information, and I went up to it and scribbled *White Coat, Black Art.*

In my commitment to live up to the show's stated purpose, I need to reveal another element that can play a small role in determining the order in which patients are seen, at least in my case. As I peruse the computer display that tracks patients in the ER, if there's no one requiring urgent care, I'm supposed to see the patient who has been waiting the longest. However, I exercise some discretion as to who I see next. I look at the nature of their problem, how long they've been waiting and, frankly, whether their case piques my interest. As midnight approached, I saw one that did just that.

11:59 P.M.

I like popping limbs back into their sockets. A patient is brought in with severe pain and an arm that doesn't work, and in two minutes, I can fix it. I feel the same way about syringing wax out of plugged ears and snaring fish bones out of throats. I love the instant gratification, not to mention the smiling face of the patient who goes home happy. Fixing dislocated shoulders can be a tricky procedure, which perhaps contributes to my interest.

A twenty-two-year-old man named Bob had been admitted an hour or so earlier with what's called an anterior glenohumeral shoulder dislocation: the ball of the humerus, a long bone that runs from the elbow to the shoulder, had been pulled out of the socket on the shoulder blade. It's one of the most common of all joint dislocations. It's easy to recognize. Ordinarily, the muscles of the shoulder girdle give it a rounded muscular appearance. When the ball of the humerus is pulled out of the socket, the shoulder takes on a squared-off look. A good emergency physician or triage nurse can spot a shoulder dislocation from across the waiting room.

Bob had been swimming when his humerus popped out of place, the second time this had happened in recent years. He was calm and respectful, as was his girlfriend, who had come in with him. I sensed he was playing it cool, acting brave and not complaining, but he must have been in considerable pain.

The method I used to put the ball of the humerus back into Bob's socket is known as the Milch technique, so named for Dr. Henry Milch, a prominent New York orthopedic surgeon who devised the procedure in 1938. Before starting I told the nurses assisting me— the manoeuvre works best with three people—to give Bob a dose of a very short-acting narcotic used to control pain Fentanyl, plus an anaesthetic called propofol or Diprivan. Anaesthetists jokingly refer to propofol as "milk of amnesia" because it's white like a laxative and it can make patients utter very wild and strange things that they have no memory of later. The drug is attractive because it takes effect almost right away and wears off fast too, leaving the patient clear-headed. It also reduces muscles spasms, making it easier to put the shoulder back in, which can require considerable brute strength. Propofol was one of the drugs that Michael Jackson took just before his death in 2009.

We had Bob sit up in the stretcher, and I bent the affected arm at the elbow and began pulling on it to create traction as I also bent and rotated the humerus away from his shoulder. I followed this by bringing the arm back and rotating it until the humerus was once again resting beside his chest and shoulder blade. As I did this, two nurses pulled his chest and shoulder blade in the opposite direction, using bedsheets placed front and back under his armpit and held behind his opposite shoulder. The idea was to separate the ball of the humerus from the lower lip of the socket of the shoulder blade. The ball is often jammed against the lower lip of the socket. If you don't separate the two, you frequently can't fix the shoulder.

When you do the Milch technique, you want to hear a click or feel a thunk that tells you the shoulder is back in place. There is no sweeter sound than a shoulder popping successfully back in. In Bob's case, it happened a moment after we began the procedure. For all the time it took fussing with the sheets, he was instantly better. As soon as the drugs wore off, a few minutes later, he was discharged and on his way home. "Let's go for a beer," he said to his girlfriend as they checked out. Not a great idea, but he was no longer my problem.

As I left Bob's bedside, I felt myself getting a groove. In emergency medicine, we're trained to expect the unexpected. Still, my colleagues and I like to think there's at least some degree of predictability to the flow of patients we see during the night shift.

Patients who are intoxicated with alcohol are most likely to arrive around 2:00 a.m., and not just because the bars have closed. Many come from home. My take on why this happens? They've sobered up enough after a night's drinking to realize something is wrong with them beyond a hangover. The booze has finally caught up with them and their liver or pancreas or heart has had enough.

The elderly who suffer from real or imagined ailments of some degree, although not necessarily life-threatening, often show up around 5:00 a.m. I think that's because they've been debating for hours whether to wait until the morning when their family doctor or specialist clocks in at work but have become too anxious to make it through the last four or five hours when the regular day begins. So they come to us as much for reassurance as for treatment.

Heart attack and stroke victims often arrive at the ER around six in the morning or an hour or so later. Virend Somers, a cardiologist at the Mayo Clinic, did a study published in the *Journal of the American Heart Association* in 2004 that reported heart attacks and strokes were 30 to 50 percent more likely to occur in the early morning than later in the day. According to Somers, the cause may be that the blood vessels that nourish the heart and the brain are less able to handle the strain in the early morning hours. Early morning heart attacks might also have something to do with an automatic surge in the stress hormone cortisol that occurs as the body prepares to wake up and face the day.

"A disproportionate number of heart attacks often occur early in the morning," says Dr. Steven Friedman, an emergency physician at Toronto Western and Toronto General hospitals. "There is a whole life cycle to the night shift. When I started years ago, you'd come on and for the first few hours you'd work like crazy, and the last few hours there would be no one registering and you'd use those few hours to clean up the backlog, and then you'd probably still have an hour or two to put your head down and sleep. I find that doesn't really happen anymore. Our emergency department shifts end at 8:00 a.m. Between 6:00 and 7:00 you'd usually have an hour of peace. Hopefully you'd cleaned up the backlog and no one [with a significant problem] had registered. But it now happens often enough—and it happened to me [recently]—that you've just finally begun to slow down . . . and have this big cardiac arrest."

Dr. Eddy Lang thinks there are two waves of patients who come to the ER during the night (apart from those who have an urgent reason, such as a car crash). "There are patients that can't sleep and come in with minor complaints between midnight and 2:00 and 3:00 a.m." he says. "And there is a group of patients who are really genuinely sick and as the evening progresses and it gets closer to midnight, they're kind of like, wow, I don't know if I'm going to make it, but I think I'll be okay until morning, whether it's a breathing problem or some kind of severe pain. And often at around 5:00 or 6:00 a.m. they realize they just can't take it anymore. We often get some really sick people first thing in the morning, just before the night shift ends. We're the last place people can go when they're looking for that kind of desperate help."

Lang especially remembers a patient in her fifties or sixties who arrived in what he would categorize as the first wave, around 2:00 a.m. "She came in complaining that she couldn't sleep because she was hearing voices," he said. "Initially when you hear that kind of story, you're thinking okay, here is a patient who is developing some psychotic symptoms and having voices speak to her. But then as I got into it deeper, it turned out she actually came to the emergency department because her neighbours had their TV on too loud. She was thinking we could help talk to her landlord or send someone in to quiet things down."

12:18 A.M.

The next patient I dealt with sent the tone of the shift in a very different direction. It was a man who thought he might have been slipped a date rape drug and sexually assaulted the evening before. Although this is not a common complaint, neither is it entirely rare. Sadly, the use of these "club drugs," so called because they tend to be added to a person's drink surreptitiously at a nightclub, has been increasing in recent years.

These drugs, of which there are several different kinds available on the street, were developed to treat an array of problems such as insomnia and clinical depression. Some are used as a general anaesthetic, especially on animals. They tend to have no colour, smell or taste (one is slightly salty) and are usually slipped into a drink and consumed without the victim being aware anything has happened. Both males and females are targeted, although it tends to happen far more to women. Once the drug takes effect, the victim can pass out or become too disoriented to resist a sexual advance. In many cases, the victim can't remember what took place once the drug kicked in or has too hazy a memory to accurately detail what occurred.

Michael was a man in his mid-thirties who arrived accompanied by his sister. He told the triage nurse he had been feeling hung-over and drowsy since having dinner with a man the night before and feared he had been drugged and possibly sexually assaulted. His life, he said, was highly stressful due to a recent death in the family. The man was a friend he had invited over for a meal. "We were not romantically involved in any way," he emphasized. "Frankly, that was the last thing on my mind. I was lonely and tired of eating on my own." His friend offered to bring dessert.

He said he did not drink any alcohol with the meal or at any other time that night. The dessert the friend provided, however, "had a slight bitter taste," but he ate it nonetheless to be polite. Not long afterwards, around 10:00 p.m., he began to feel uncon-trollably sleepy and needed to go to bed. As he stumbled into the bedroom, he thought he might have been drugged. At some point in the night or in the early morning, he remembered waking up to find the man in bed with him. "I felt his presence and then I must have fallen right back to sleep," he said. "The next thing I knew it was about 11:00 a.m. and I was alone in bed." It was most uncom-mon for him, he added, to sleep for seven hours a night, never mind thirteen. Since waking up he had battled a need to go back to sleep, which was again not normal.

The nurse observed no obvious signs of distress, although

Michael was a bit anxious, a typical reaction for someone telling a difficult, if not traumatic, story. Michael appeared to be alert and was walking normally, but he said he still felt drowsy and hungover. He did not complain of a headache or any obvious neurological symptoms. His vital signs were all within the normal range, he didn't have a temperature and his Glasgow Coma Scale (GCS) score was 15, or totally normal.

The GCS was developed by two professors of neurosurgery at the University of Glasgow in the 1970s primarily to determine the level of consciousness in head injury victims; it's a way to assess a patient's conscious state. The higher the number, the more awake the patient. Any rating below 9 is not good, and likely means the patient is deeply unconscious. Someone who arrives with a mild head injury would probably have a GCS of about 14.

To someone schooled in the typical date rape potions, Michael's story had a significant red flag. None of the typical drugs has a bitter taste, as he reported. A defence lawyer would likely focus any criminal case, if he decided to charge the man, on that factor. But my long-standing interest in prescription drug abuse made me think there was an explanation that lent credibility to what he reported. There was, in fact, a smoking gun.

From research, I knew about a fairly new group of drugs known as Z-hypnotics—Zopiclone (also sold under the name Lunesta), Zolpidem and Zaleplon—that are nighttime sedatives used to treat insomnia.

Following the rampant misuse of OxyContin, the U.S. Food and Drug Administration (FDA) had enacted regulations requiring all new generic narcotics coming on the market to have a risk management program designed to help physicians and pharmacists identify people who might be at risk of abusing the drugs. I was retained as a consultant to develop educational materials for certain pharmaceutical clients. One of the drugs I worked on was Zopiclone. Part of my research required me to pore over reports on any adverse side effects of Zopiclone/Lunesta. As the saying goes, if I had a dollar for every time dysgeusia—bitter taste in the mouth—was listed as a side effect I would be writing this from a private island in a perpetually warm locale. I also knew that a high dosage of Zopiclone could cause somnolence, the state of feeling drowsy sometimes to the point of exhaustion. There is a moment after you take Zopiclone when you feel an uncontrollable need to fall asleep. It comes on so quickly you don't know what hit you.

A little bell went off in my head as I pieced together Michael's story and my knowledge of the Z-hypnotics. My gut told me the friend had slipped a certain number of crushed-up pills, likely Zopiclone, into the dessert, and then taken advantage of Michael to some degree in bed. There were no obvious signs of sexual penetration, but sexual assault can encompass many other forms.

Although I believed Michael—and a physician's code says we are supposed to align ourselves with our patients unless there's evidence they're lying—proving what he said would require hard evidence. The tests I'd ordered found no alcohol in his blood, which corroborated his story. But our lab at Mount Sinai wasn't set up to detect Zopiclone. The Hospital for Sick Children, located directly across the street from Mount Sinai, did have that capacity. I sent Michael's blood there and asked them to test for it.

Unfortunately, a few days after I sent the blood to Sick Kids, I learned belatedly that Zopiclone cannot be tested through blood; it requires a sample of urine. I didn't know this, nor did the attending nurse. Should I have? Perhaps. But there are new drugs coming on the market all the time. It's impossible to keep up with the torrent of information that flows across our desks and into our computers every month. By the time I found out we needed a urine sample, it was far too late to test Michael, as all traces of the drug had long since disappeared from his body.

What, then, could I do for him? Perhaps I provided him with the most important service we could, which was to validate what he had told us. We tried to be supportive. At the very least, I didn't want to retraumatize him.

All of us in the ER have some things we do better than others. I believe one thing that I do well is to listen extra hard to people who are experiencing social and psychological trauma. When I encounter someone like Michael, the last thing I want to do is to make him feel worse about what he's gone through. I think my empathy, if I can claim to have that, stems from my own insecurities, and from my own need to be listened to and believed.

While I believed Michael's story, I don't always accept that a patient is telling the truth. In fact, I think many either lie or misrepresent the facts of their case to me and the other professionals at the ER who treat them.

There have been countless books written about lying. Dr. Michael Lewis of the Robert Wood Johnson Medical School in New Jersey, co-author of *Lying and Deception in Everyday Life,* has conducted extensive research on the subject. "In a single day, most people lie a minimum of 25 times," he estimates.

The online service called WebMD.com conducted a survey in 2004 that asked readers the question: "Do you lie to your doctor?" Approximately half of the 1,500 respondents admitted they did. The survey didn't focus on encounters with ER doctors, but the results are interesting nonetheless. WebMD found that younger people, those between the ages of twenty-five and thirty-four, tend to lie more than people over fifty-five. Males and females lied about the same amount except when it came to one question: "How much do you drink?" Males were more likely to report a far lower amount than was true. Both sexes claimed they were good at deception, with doctors catching them in a lie less than 10 percent of the time, or at least that's what they wanted to believe. I'm guessing the doctors knew the patients were fibbing far more often than they realized.

The most common things they lied about were no surprise: following their doctor's orders, exercising, smoking, their sexual habits, and alcohol and drug use. Six percent said they lied about their personal or family history. Only 2 percent said they didn't tell a doctor about all of their symptoms.

I found the reasons why people lied to their doctor noteworthy. The most common by far, at 50 percent, was that they "didn't want to be judged." This suggests to me that a doctor would be wise to know how he or she acts and reacts as a patient explains his medical history and symptoms. A patient, for example, could interpret an arched eyebrow at the wrong moment as disapproval.

The next most likely reason was a fear that the truth would be "just too embarrassing." A patient's personal makeup is probably the primary determining factor in his comfort level when talking about certain matters, but again, medical staff can help or hinder this kind of communication. Let's say I sensed a female patient was not at ease discussing certain personal matters with me. I could ask a female doctor or resident or nurse to take over some of the discussion. Better to get the information than worry about my ego.

The third and only other significant factor that led to lying, at more than 30 percent, was a perception that "the doctor wouldn't understand." I'm not clear as to what would cause that perception. It's possible a bored or impatient response on our part might contribute. Or perhaps the young people who responded to the survey just felt that way in general about doctors, who were likely much older than them—like me.

I think, however, that the respondents left out what I consider one of the main reasons patients lie to doctors: because they lie to themselves. They don't necessarily want to confront the inconvenient truths of their lives.

It was no surprise to me that lying about drinking was prevalent. We deal with a lot of people with alcohol issues at the ER. Sadly, alcohol is a huge contributor to everything from organ malfunctions to every kind of accident. It's important to get a sense of how much patients consume. I know they might not tell me their actual consumption amount, but I want to get as close to the truth as I can. I've learned the best way to do this is not by asking patients if they are alcoholics, which sounds judgmental. And they will probably say, "No, I'm not." Instead, I ask how much they drink on an average day, a question that relates more to what they consider to be normal behaviour. If they hang out with people who knock back six or seven beers on a daily basis, and they drink only three or four a day, they'll see their own consumption as moderate. But three or four drinks a day meets the criteria for substance abuse or problem drinking.

Another self-deception has to do with sexual activity. I can't tell you how many times I have had female patients come in with what was obviously genital herpes and claim to have no idea what it was or how they acquired it. Fair enough. That can happen. But once diagnosed, they continue to deny that it could be a sexually transmitted disease. One twenty-year-old checked in with pain around her vulva, which was red and covered with a smattering of blisters. Her lymph nodes were tender and she was feeling unwell. These are classic symptoms of a herpes outbreak. I told her I was certain about my diagnosis.

"It's not possible," she said. "I have a boyfriend. We don't sleep around."

Her personal life was not my business. But if she had genital herpes I had to notify the department of public health. "They'll need to know all your sexual partners and your boyfriend's," I said. When I told her this she froze. Then she became angry and accused me of jumping to a false conclusion. To calm her down, I told one of my twenty-five lies of that day. "Maybe you're right," I said. "It could be something else." I then offered to break a blister, swab it and have it analyzed. "Then we'll know for sure."

I could see in her eyes that she knew what the results would prove. "Is it possible," she asked, "that my boyfriend could have herpes and not know it?"

I thought she had gone through enough of a shock for one day, so I told another lie, albeit one that had a half sliver of a chance of being true. "Maybe he never knew he had primary herpes and one day he had a reoccurrence, had a sore [which would need to be present for her to contract the herpes; if there's no outbreak the virus can't be transmitted], and wasn't aware of what it was," I said. She nodded almost imperceptibly. This version she could handle. I didn't think for a second that he didn't know. A genital herpes outbreak is not something you can pass off as a minor rash. It weakens your system considerably, sometimes to the point where you get a fever and the shakes; it demands your attention.

As she waited for the news that would change her life forever, I felt sorry for the young woman. My instinct told me her boyfriend had passed the virus on to her uncaringly, although that was pure conjecture on my part. It made me angry. I see so much suffering in my job that when the pain, in this case both physical and emotional, could have easily been avoided (people with herpes can have an active sex life as long as they refrain during outbreaks), it sometimes fills me with quiet rage.

———————

I was filling out my paperwork on Michael's case when my resident came in to tell me the medical history of several patients she had been dealing with. Before she began I asked her about the CT scan for Curtis. He was the patient with the possible appendicitis who was enduring the long wait outside my office with his mother and his antsy wife.

"Oh my God," she said. "I completely forgot about it." The results had been waiting for her on the X-ray reporting system for at least two hours. Instead of chastising the resident, I told her about the many times I had forgotten about patients myself. In our overburdened health care system, we tend to respond to crises. She had been focusing on patients with more immediate needs.

When the resident retrieved the CT, we saw that Curtis did not have appendicitis. It was likely just a case of heartburn. I shouldn't have felt this way, but I was conflicted about the outcome. I was glad Curtis was fine, but I knew his wife would be even more steamed that the wait had been for nothing.

I was right. "All this wasted time out here," she said, indicating the hallways and glaring at me with cold eyes. Curtis and his mother were nicer and just seemed relieved that the news was good and they could now go home. I decided it might be best not to mention that the results had been available a while ago. I didn't lie. I just didn't volunteer the information. A night shift in the ER is hard enough without adding avoidable conflict. I apologized for their inconvenience and moved on.

CHAPTER FOUR

FEAR AND LOATHING

12:47 A.M.

Two police detectives were waiting for me near the main triage desk; one was a tall male in a sleek black suit, probably in his early forties. He was ruggedly handsome in the manner of Jean-Paul Belmondo, the French actor who played a slew of cops and criminals during his long film career. His partner was a decade or so younger, thin and pretty with long blond hair. Her crisp blouse and grey skirt suggested a TV reporter more than a cop.

They introduced themselves and told me they were investigating two incidents that had taken place a few hours earlier in a trendy part of the city. One of the victims was a fifteen-year-old white male who had been swarmed by a gang of South Asian teenagers in what the police thought might be a racially motivated crime. The boy's father, after being called by his injured son on his cellphone, had brought him to Mount Sinai. The other victim, around the same age, had been injured and was being treated at another hospital in the north end of the city. The detectives wanted me to examine the boy right away so they could interview him when I was finished.

"We think the attacks are related," the female detective said. "This gang has a history of going down to the area and picking fights with the white kids down there. It's been happening for a while."

I agreed to see the young man next. He was big for his age, as so many are these days. At almost six feet tall and close to 200 pounds, he looked older than his years. He had a bad laceration about three centimetres long on the back of his leg, and some minor bruises on his face. I asked him what had happened.

"I was with my cousin out on the street near a coffee shop where we hang out when a fight broke out not far from us," he said. "I didn't want any part of it because I was with her so we started to walk away. A few minutes later a whole bunch of them ran at us. They were punching me and I curled up to protect myself and then someone hit me on the back of the leg with something. Maybe a bat or an iron bar. I don't know."

Our focus as doctors is on the injuries themselves and on the mechanism of the injuries, not on the "he said, she said." My primary purpose was to get the boy talking so I could establish his mental alertness and (of course) so I could check his leg.

He was lucid and calm and able to follow the movement of my finger as I passed it vertically and horizontally in front of him. I assessed him as 15 on the Glasgow Coma Scale. There was a faint smell of ethanol on his breath.

"Why do you think they attacked you?"

"I don't know," he said. "Maybe they think we're all rich snobs or something. Because of where we live."

"We're not rich, I can tell you that, and we got no prejudice," his father interjected. "Maybe some other kids ain't nice to them."

The boy wanted me to patch him up so he could go home. I was fine to do that—a few sutures would do the trick.

I asked if they were okay to talk to the detectives; they consented. I left the room and let the police know they could come in.

"What did he tell you?" the male detective asked.

"That he was willing to talk to you," I said. I tried to look pleasant and hoped he'd get the implicit message: ask the patient what you like, but don't pressure me to divulge anything a patient has told me. On a busy emergency shift, when I'm running from patient to patient, it's all I can do to keep focused on patient care. Anything beyond that often feels like it's taking me from my main duty. The last thing I want to do is have an argument with a detective about what I can and cannot reveal.

A little slit of a smile creased his face as he led his partner into the patient's room. He knew all too well I was under no obligation to reveal anything whatsoever to him, but he had tried nonetheless. I didn't blame him, and he accepted my response in a polite and professional way. It was his job to ask and mine to refuse. The two detectives had been around for a while and understood the rules. Some of the younger officers, however, can be more aggressive about pressing for information. Either they are ignorant of the boundaries or they just don't care.

Hospital workers are not agents of the police. We are legally obligated to inform them if someone comes in with a gunshot wound, but not if it's a knife wound or a beating from a fight. We don't have to tell them any details of a case, especially the results of a tox screen that could contain alcohol or drug levels. If they want that information they need to get a warrant—or in the case of alcohol, do their own breath test.

On the other hand, if we suspect a child has been abused we must inform the Children's Aid Society. However, if we suspect a woman has suffered a domestic assault (or a man, for that matter), we are not required to report it. If victims wish to press charges, that's their right. But we're far more concerned with the patient's personal welfare than with a possible police complaint. We ask a social worker to see the patients so that they know their options. Even if they decide it's safe to go home, we counsel them to have an emergency plan of escape that includes at least a packed overnight bag and a few dollars hidden away in case they have to leave home abruptly.

There was one instance, however, when I decided I had to intervene whether the victim wanted me to or not. Many years ago at another hospital, paramedics wheeled in a twenty-two-year-old woman who was in a semi-conscious state, accompanied by her husband. She had a broken nose and bruised ribs. A CT scan of her head revealed a subdural hematoma that required a neurosurgical operation to remove a clot.

It was obvious she had been beaten, and I had a pretty good idea her husband was responsible. He was short, and I sensed from the way he tried to puff out his chest that he tried to overcompensate for his lack of height. His physique was wiry, and he had a menacing air that made me uncomfortable. This was not someone you'd like to cross.

He acted solicitous and feigned concern for his wife, but it didn't seem genuine. I asked him how she became injured, and he said she had slipped on something in the kitchen. After each of my questions he glared at me in a manner I found intimidating. He seemed coiled, ready to spring at the slightest provocation.

After the paramedics came to transfer the woman to the hospital where she would be seen by a neurosurgeon, I called the police and told them my suspicions. I was worried that she might not survive the next beating: in these types of relationships another assault is usually a given. The police said someone would go to the hospital and investigate. I never knew the outcome, but I hope she had the courage to press charges. However, having just tasted a small dose of the intimidation she probably lived under all the time, I would have understood whatever decision she made.

———————————

Another of my cases that involved the police arose after a twenty-something male came in with a laceration on the joint near a knuckle on his right hand. He told me he had fallen, but his injury was not consistent with that type of accident. I suspected he had been in a fight, which meant he could have been cut by human teeth.

"You need to tell me what happened," I said. "If it was from someone's teeth and the germs from their mouth got into your hand, they could cause a severe infection that could destroy the joints and the tendons. The wound has to be irrigated and possibly examined in the OR."

"Let's just say that you should do what you need to do in case, you know, hypothetically there was a fight," he said.

It so happened that at the same time this patient arrived, another young male was admitted with a broken nose and some broken teeth. He told the triage nurse he had been punched in the mouth and was considering pressing charges. He also mentioned that he had seen the person who had struck him being admitted to the ER, and had called the police.

Two constables arrived soon after, and once they heard that the alleged perpetrator might be in another room they started pressuring the nurse in charge to tell them where he was. She refused even to confirm that the alleged perpetrator was there. A tense stand-off ensued. I stepped in to support the nurse. The police constable was clearly trying to intimidate her. He even threatened to have her charged with obstruction of justice.

On the one hand, as ER doctors and nurses, we are trained to be helpful. If patients look as if they need medical assistance or seem to be in distress, we're programmed to assist however we can. When the police want information, there's an instinct that says we should co-operate by telling them what they want to know. After all, they help us. I can't tell you how many times over the years we've had to call the police to restrain a patient who has suddenly gone berserk. And we're awfully glad when an officer accompanies an intoxicated patient to the ER for stitches before taking him away on an assault charge.

In rural emergency departments, the relationship between ER staff and law enforcement is even more symbiotic. In my time, smaller hospitals maintained a skeleton security staff at night. If a patient suddenly became violent, ER staff called on the local detachment of the Ontario Provincial Police to help restrain the patient. A kind of coziness can develop between the police and ER staff. It's not uncommon for an ER nurse to invite officers to help themselves to the goodies we put out at night. I've also heard of police bringing doughnuts to the emergency department.

Then there's the power of the police to intimidate all of us— not just ER doctors and nurses. When we're driving, police have the power to make us pull over and show them our driver's licence, proof of insurance, and vehicle ownership. You can't tell me some of that feeling of intimidation doesn't come into play the moment a police constable asks about a patient.

On the other hand, there's the duty to protect patient confidentiality, a principle as old as the Hippocratic Oath, and one that weighs heavily on my mind as I write these pages. Not surprisingly, many of the doctors and the nurses who work in the ER get more than a little unnerved when asked about patients by police officers. When you're on duty and focused on patient care, it's hard to keep all the rules and the exceptions regarding confidentiality in your mind. If you tell the police what they want to know, will you be sued by the patient or charged with professional misconduct later on? Charges aside, what will patients think of you if it turns out that under pressure you squawked like a nervous parrot when you didn't have to?

I stepped in between the nurse and the police constable because I could sense it was one of those moments when the rules were more grey than black and white. My primary purpose, though, was to support my nursing colleague. I too refused to reveal medical information. I confirmed that the other man was in the ER but agreed that the nurse had been correct not to release any patient information. I told the police they were not allowed to speak to the man while he was being treated but they were welcome to wait until he was released, which they chose to do. The nurse and I chatted privately afterwards. She said she was glad I had backed her up. I told her I admired her guts for standing up to a police constable who was trying (and succeeding) to intimidate her. In case you're wondering, the nurse in question had already summoned hospital security to make certain the alleged victim, and any bystanders in the ER, were safe.

I don't want you to think we're always high and mighty when it comes to patient confidentiality. Health professionals, being human, love to dish gossip. And there's nothing more delicious than the medical secrets of patients, especially famous ones.

Michael Jackson, the self-proclaimed "King of Pop," was pronounced dead following a cardiac arrest at UCLA Medical Center on June 25, 2009, at 2:26 p.m., Los Angeles time. At 2:44 p.m., a scant eighteen minutes later, TMZ.com broke the news on its gossip website. It's been called the celebrity scoop of the decade. The third paragraph of the story posted to TMZ.com is as follows: "A source tells us Jackson was dead when paramedics arrived. A cardiologist at UCLA tells TMZ Jackson died of cardiac arrest." Two paragraphs later, the following is written: "A source inside the hospital told us there was 'absolute chaos' after Jackson arrived. People who were with the singer were screaming, 'You've got to save him! You've got to save him!'"

The tense final moments in Michael Jackson's life were probably filled with frantic efforts to revive him. I can tell you that when a person, famous or otherwise, is brought to the resuscitation room in full cardiac arrest, the doors are closed, the curtains are pulled, and the team of ER doctors, nurses, anaesthetists, cardiologists, and respiratory therapists goes to work. Aside from the (growing number of) family members who wish to remain present, no one else is allowed in the room.

The point is that it's highly likely that TMZ.com was able to break the news of Michael Jackson's death because a health professional bound by confidentiality broke that oath. I think that breach was wrong, and whoever leaked the information should face repercussions from the governing California medical bodies.

It's not just famous people who are gossiped about by medical staff. In November 2002, three Toronto researchers conducted a study to examine patient confidentiality in the real world of medicine.

They recruited five medical students to ride the elevators at St. Michael's Hospital, a busy tertiary-care hospital in downtown Toronto that is affiliated with the University of Toronto's faculty of medicine. The students were instructed to listen to and record any conversation among medical personnel in which patient confidentiality was violated.

The students reported that, over the two-week period of the study, hospital caregivers made eighteen comments that violated patient confidentiality on thirteen of 113 elevator rides. On some of the rides, more than one confidentiality violation was observed. Interestingly, doctors were the worst offenders; eleven of the eighteen comments were made by MDs. Most referred to patients by their initials or by the reason for their admission to hospital. In four instances, the name of the patient was used.

The study was published in the venerable *British Medical Journal* on November 1, 2003. The authors noted that the study strengthened "the evidence that public lapses in patient confidentiality are widespread."

Many of us use "code" to talk about patients within earshot of bystanders. I've heard one resident say this to a colleague on another service: "That ischemic bowel on our service is circling the drain [likely to die]." Substituting the name of the disease for the name of the patient may still be a violation of privacy if the patient's disease or circumstances are very rare or unusual.

The point is, we're both trained and inclined to do the right thing, but sometimes we slip up. I told the police the suspect was in the ER because I thought it was the right thing to do. I believe that having to remain silent is one of the reasons why health professionals tend to bottle up their feelings. In my opinion, our professional culture encourages and often compels us to remain silent on so many matters that it contributes to rampant rates of burnout among physicians, nurses and other health professionals.

Patient confidentiality, and all the rules governing it, is without question an essential aspect of the ethical framework under which we operate. But it is not an absolute. Common sense, as well as the emotional health of medical professionals, should also dictate whether we share certain information. At times we need to talk about what we see and do. It's not healthy to repress the often volatile feelings we experience. But remaining silent and stoic is seen as the optimum way a medical professional should function. I think there has to be a way for us to respect all the confidential information we possess that at the same time allows us to vent and process what we need to get out in the open. I'm not always sure the powers that be agree.

————————

My interactions with the police at Mount Sinai have thankfully been isolated, because few victims of violent crime are brought to our ER. One other case does stand out, however, because I eventually had to testify about it in court.

It began on the early evening of June 7, 2006. The police arrived at the ER with twenty-four-year-old Shayne Fisher, whom they had arrested during a drug raid at a known crack den earlier in the day. He had been visiting a friend, a drug trafficker named Steve Ruiz. When seven police officers broke into the high-rise apartment to execute a search warrant, they arrested Ruiz, Fisher and another man. Fisher was charged with a firearms offence, which he denied. Ruiz later told police he had thrown three firearms over the balcony as the police stormed in and that none of them belonged to the other two men.

When I treated Fisher, he told me the police had beaten him up even though he hadn't resisted arrest. I noted several significant injuries, which turned out to be a fractured rib, a perforated right eardrum and bruising around the right eye. The police said he had fallen down a flight of stairs. It looked to me like he had taken a beating.

About two years later, I testified at Fisher's trial before Ontario

Superior Court Justice Brian Trafford. I detailed the injuries I had observed and estimated, conservatively, that Fisher had received at least four blows consistent with his claim that he had been roughed up. Justice Trafford accepted Fisher's version of what had happened, dismissed the firearms charges against him and his friend and called the testimony of the drug squad officers "unreliable [and] likely false." Ruiz, for the record, had pleaded guilty to the drug and weapons charges against him.

While Mount Sinai sees a scant number of crime victims or perpetrators—sometimes they are one and the same—there are hospitals where it's a common occurrence, especially in large U.S. cities. Dr. Bruce Campana, who has been an emergency physician at Vancouver General Hospital since the early 1990s, spent his residency at Denver General County Hospital from 1984 to 1987. "We called it the gun and knife club," he says, adding that it was a great hospital that found a way to function well on a limited budget. "The place was a zoo, indescribable. We had a full jail with armed guards in the hospital. The hallways were always full of patients and half the time they were handcuffed to the beds. As soon as you finished with one trauma patient and got them off to the OR there would be another one."

One episode that occurred in the middle of the night remains forever in his memory. "They brought this bad guy in who had a gunshot wound to the head from another bad guy," he says. "He needed to be intubated using a laryngoscope. Before that happened he immediately vomited on me. I was dripping with his vomit and smelling like Italian food and wine. From the corner of my eye I saw a man coming in with something metal in his hand. I thought to myself, thank God anaesthesia is here to help me intubate this guy. Then out of every corner of the department these police officers and armed guards jump on this guy. It wasn't an anaesthesiologist with a laryngoscope; it was the other bad guy with a gun coming to finish off and kill the man I was working on, perhaps me as well. That guy was taken away in this blur of blue uniforms and I never saw him again. My guy died from the gunshot wound."

Another Canadian emergency physician who spent time in the U.S. is Dr. Ronald Stewart. A member of the Order of Canada and the former minister of health in Nova Scotia, Stewart is also known for having been a script consultant on two prominent American TV shows, *Emergency!* and *Marcus Welby, M.D.*, much earlier in his career. Those opportunities arose when Stewart moved to Los Angeles in 1972 after surviving a horrific accident. It was 3:00 a.m. during a snowstorm in northern Cape Breton, and Stewart was out on a house call when his car plunged over a cliff near Neil's Harbour. He suffered a severe brain injury that almost killed him.

Following a painful recovery period, Stewart decided to radically change his life. The twenty-nine-year-old applied for a residency at the University of Southern California County General and was chosen over fifty-nine other applicants. He packed his Volvo and drove for five days from Neil's Harbour to Los Angeles. "I had never seen a wound intentionally done by someone else. I had never seen a drug addict," he says. "When I arrived I was on surgery the next day. In that shift I admitted five patients with stab wounds and four gunshot wounds. My job as an emergency resident was to keep them alive while the surgeons were operating in the OR, and assisting occasionally depending on how bad it got."

It often got very bad. "The hospital was in the middle of a ghetto, on the border of two big gangs," Stewart says. "Every Friday night the gangs would get in a big brawl and they would shoot and stab each other and come to us. [One time] we had a gun battle in the emergency department. That was scary. I was bagging a patient [using an inflatable bag to pump oxygen into his lungs]. He had been shot in the head. We were intubating him, squeezing

the bag under the stretcher, feeling his pulse with the other hand."
The man soon died, and when another resident went to the waiting
room where various members from both gangs and their families
had gathered, an intense gunfight erupted. "I was cowering under
the stretcher," Stewart says. "It resulted in a lot of changes to security at the hospital. Now they have metal detectors. It's sad."

Stewart was also exposed to some of the darker aspects of the
human condition. "I was in Los Angeles for eight years and there is
every perversion known to mankind in L.A., truly. The most bizarre
would be self-mutilation," he says. "We would have patients come in
holding a body part and asking me, 'Can you fix this?' We had several in a row that had biblical allusions, biblical references. One was
found by a paramedic sitting at his kitchen table reading from the
Bible the passages: 'If thine eye offend thee, pluck it out' and 'If thy
right hand offend thee, cut it off,' which he promptly did. Because
he cut off his hand he couldn't reach his eye. That was the call I got
on the radio. I thought it was a joke at first but it wasn't. There were
several cases of sexual mutilation. Self-castration was not unusual.
I learned that the human mind can make people do tremendously
harmful things."

The hospital had a jail ward on the thirteenth floor that was
run by the medical residents. "The rules were that when you were
arrested for a misdemeanour and were injured, which happened frequently, or were suspected of having [swallowed] illicit drugs, or
[were going through] a drug overdose, you went to the jail ward,"
says Stewart. "Every morning there was a parade from the big bus
that came from the jail that would pull up to our emergency department. They would walk prisoners, chained legs and arms, through
the department to the elevator to the jail ward. That was despite the
fact in the parking garage underneath the hospital the elevator was
right there. They could have loaded them there. That was part of

the punishment, I guess. I complained to the administration. It was cruel and unusual punishment to have them publicly humiliated in that way. I lost that battle easily."

One of the prisoners who came to the jail ward was serial killer Charles Manson, who was often injured in fights in prison. Known for his wild eyes, which, Stewart says, would "look right through you," Manson found his nemesis in the head nurse. "She was tough as nails, with a wonderful kind and soft heart, but she could look severe," says Stewart. "She was the first person who could stare Charles Manson down. He turned his eyes away when she stared at him."

Stewart left L.A. in 1979 to become the founding head of the emergency medicine department at the University of Pittsburgh. While in the Steel City he became the central character in a dramatic and terrifying rescue that was worthy of a Hollywood film. An ironworker who was helping to demolish a bridge in Pittsburgh had both his legs trapped and crushed when a section of the bridge unexpectedly shifted. Stewart was summoned to try and free the man, who was pinned near the top of the tall structure. "I had to climb the [fire] ladder and it was 130 feet above the river," he says. "I remember looking down [and seeing] a big police boat with a big net below. I was thinking, oh my, this doesn't look good."

Several paramedics had already reached the worker and, on Stewart's instructions, hooked up IV lines, including one that administered morphine to help the man deal with his excruciating pain. It took three hours for the emergency rescue team to extricate one of the man's legs. "We found that the vertical strut holding up the bridge was impaling his other leg and we couldn't cut it away with the acetylene torch," he says. At this point there were six people high above the water, including Stewart and the patient. The bridge suddenly shifted a few inches and they feared it might soon collapse. The only solution was to amputate the trapped leg as quickly as possible, which Stewart did successfully. It was such a noteworthy case that he wrote about it in the *Journal of Trauma*.

While that kind of life-threatening danger is rare for an ER physician, there is always some element of risk in each shift, as some of the people who end up in the emergency ward are not mentally stable. My next patient reminded me of that potential.

1:15 A.M.

I had heard the loud ranting ever since the paramedics had brought in Pat, as I will call him, an hour or so earlier. It was impossible to avoid his caterwauling even though the door to his room was tightly shut. Pat had been talking gibberish non-stop at a high volume since his arrival. In his early to mid-thirties, Pat was wearing, of all things, a tuxedo. He was either not able, or not willing, to answer any questions my resident posed to him. He had no identification on him nor was he someone we knew from a previous encounter.

A few weeks earlier I had had another disturbed patient who was virtually catatonic except for one phrase he repeated no matter what he was asked.

"Do you know your name, sir?" I asked the man, who was maybe in his early sixties, as he lay on a gurney facing a hospital wall.

"Fuck you," he replied in a soft voice.

"Do you know where you are?"

"Fuck you."

"Do you know what month it is?"

"Fuck you."

No matter what I asked that was his answer. He seemed fine, medically, and wasn't causing any trouble. Maybe he was just worn down by life, I thought, as I made my notes. Don't most of us, at some point, feel like saying fuck you, or something similar, when we have no energy left to communicate?

Pat, on the other hand, was physically agitated and had to be strapped on his back to a bed with leather restraints on his arms and legs to keep him from running amok in the ward. A security guard was assigned to sit outside his room, just in case he broke free. I have seen psychotic patients of small stature—females included—exhibit feats of strength that would seem impossible for someone their size. We never take chances with our safety around seemingly disturbed patients. It may be an apocryphal story, but I have heard of a short, wizened man who required eight people in the ER to restrain him. I once had to deal with a delusional man who was the size of a football lineman. He had not displayed any outward signs of aggression, so I found myself alone with him in an examination room. Psychotic people, however, can switch from passive to agitated without warning. At one point with Pat I sensed this was going to happen— he stood up and claimed I was not a certified doctor—so I made an excuse and left to get a security guard. Fortunately, Pat calmed down as soon as he saw the uniformed show of force.

Dr. Bruce Campana once feared for his life from the most unlikely patient. He was treating a small wisp of a girl for a psychiatric problem. "I thought I could charm her," he said, referring to the way he planned to gain her trust and get her to speak about her troubles. They were alone in a patient room and she was walking around, which was not unusual, when suddenly, "She picked up a pencil, turned around and came towards me," he says. "I remember thinking, 'Holy shit, she's going to plunge that pencil into [me]. I am not a martial artist and if she has a lucky stab I'm going to the operating room.' I remember being quite frightened. I made it clear that I would defend myself. She dropped the pencil and ran out of the emergency department. It was a lesson to me that big hulking guys are not always the ones that hurt you."

Although I'm cautious around potentially psychotic patients, it takes a lot for me to get truly rattled. I've dealt with so many over the years that I no longer let them get to me, although some are experts at goading staff. Dr. Pat Croskerry, who works in the ER at the Cobequid Multi-Service Centre about ten miles outside of Halifax, has been on the receiving end of numerous taunts, as have I.

Croskerry received his PhD in psychology before becoming a physician. He says that people who have what is termed borderline personality disorder (BPD) can be particularly difficult to deal with. They tend to exhibit a variety of mood swings. They usually have self-image problems and difficulty with interpersonal communication. It's hard for them to maintain effective relationships at home, at work or in social settings.

"They are not schizophrenic or bipolar or have any other disorder. They have bad personalities and the bad behaviours that go along with that," he says. "The textbook in emergency medicine says you can diagnose a borderline disorder because they tend to alienate the emergency department in the first five minutes. The expression is that they 'have PhDs in how to upset people.' They seem to be able to seize upon someone's vulnerabilities and exploit them. If you are slightly overweight, for example, they might refer to you as a fat lump. If you are on the short side they might refer to you as a midget. If you are soft-spoken and have a gentle manner they might refer to you as a homosexual. They seem to be able to exaggerate your features to upset you. They are very good at it. The death rate among these people is high. Their chance of successfully committing suicide by age thirty or forty is one in five. It is a lethal disorder."

Because someone with BPD is usually rude and obnoxious toward the nurses and physicians, the staff sometimes can't see beyond the behaviour. "When they call people names and they are violent, it has a visceral effect on [staff's] emotions and you can become aroused against the patient," Croskerry says. "That is a very dangerous position to be in—when your feelings get involved in decision making. For example, I am fairly soft-spoken and reasonably gentle with people. One of them called me a 'raving queer' just on that basis. I am quite definitely heterosexual. But if you have any reservations about yourself and you are slightly overweight and somebody calls you a fat lump, as they do, even though it is unreasonable and you can rationalize it, it nevertheless hurts. Once physicians and nurses have been hurt by these barbs and insults, they don't provide very good care. It is extremely difficult to disassociate yourself from the immediate situation and [see that] their behaviour *is* the illness. That is the mistake we make—being judgmental about them. But I must disassociate myself from my feelings the patient is eliciting. It is one of the most difficult things we must do."

Croskerry witnessed the fallout from this attitude toward BPD patients while working at Halifax's main emergency department. A huge commotion accompanied a teenage male who was being brought in on a stretcher. He was belligerent, calling people names and swearing. After a while, a nurse asked Croskerry to examine the patient. "He's a real piece of work," she said in a derogatory tone. "That's the problem with the youth today. We allow them to behave like this. None of them gets proper parenting. If I had a child like this I would wash his mouth out with soap."

It was obvious to Croskerry that the nurse held the young man in contempt and had probably not dealt with him the way she would a typical patient. Croskerry examined the patient, which was difficult as he was shoving and swinging at people and swearing profusely.

The staff managed to get an IV into his arm, which allowed them to give him a sedative. "I thought it was a drug overdose or the kid had got into ecstasy," Croskerry says. Nevertheless, he ordered a CT scan of the head. The kid, who was about sixteen or seventeen, died while the scan was taking place. It emerged afterwards that he had been out on his bicycle when a car struck him. His helmet flew off and his head landed hard on the ground. The blow to his head had caused his antics. "He was a model student with straight As. He did volunteer work around the city."

The nurse, who hadn't bothered to check with the paramedics, had discovered none of these details. "This kid was framed [on the part of the nurse] by his behaviour, which you just should not do," says Croskerry. "I'll never forget the case."

We have several BPD patients who show up regularly at Mount Sinai. Alan is one of the most problematic. About forty-two, he is five foot nothing and weighs about eighty pounds, yet is surprisingly muscular and strong. He's a diabetic who also takes a medication called Epival (known generically as valproic acid), an anticonvulsant often used to control seizures. He emits loud, terrifying sounds that unnerve other patients and their family members and friends, who assume he is either in horrific pain and is being neglected by us or is being tortured by the medical staff. At times he will throw furniture and create as much overall havoc as he can. Not surprisingly, Alan has often been admitted to a nearby psychiatric hospital that provides, among other services, a locked ward for people considered a danger to themselves or others.

Alan has one more distinguishing feature to his background; he is a transgender individual. Born a woman, he was surgically altered into a man.

One time Alan arrived at Mount Sinai at 1:00 a.m. in the company of four police officers in flak jackets and bulletproof vests and at least half a dozen security guards. About ten people hovered around him, an entourage he clearly enjoyed having summoned. I had asked the charge nurse not to triage him (begin the process of admitting him to the ER) but to keep him in the waiting room until I was free to look him over.

Our department has developed a protocol for dealing with patients who demonstrate a pattern of repeatedly tying up precious resources for reasons that almost always turn out to be unfounded. We state that we're ready and willing to treat any emergency problem, but that failing to cooperate in the absence of an obvious clinical problem will result in the patient being asked to leave the department.

My instinct that early morning told me there was nothing medically wrong with Alan, but I had to examine him nonetheless. I couldn't take a chance that he might actually be in need of care, as had often been the case in the past. On this occasion, Alan vacillated between periods of calm and intermittent screaming. The waiting room was packed, and Alan's performance was distracting and disturbing for everyone.

He greeted me by name, having established an ongoing relationship with most of the ER staff. One of Alan's ploys was to insert drill bits into his surgically-fashioned member, a habit for which one of the nurses had dubbed Alan "Tool Guy." This kind of behaviour was hardly unique. I have met patients with BPD who have inserted pencils, kitchen utensils and even razor blades into various orifices of the body. One woman I looked after at another hospital claimed to have swallowed such objects even when she hadn't, which tended to elicit sympathy from the paramedics (if they hadn't dealt with her before) and the police officers. On the occasions when she was telling the truth, she was usually able to pass the pencil through in a bowel movement. If the object had become impacted in her stomach, she needed to have it removed through an endoscope or in the operating room. She had also inserted many a sharp object into her vagina, and had ingested large doses of prescription drugs, enough at times to qualify as an overdose.

One thing about Alan; I got the impression he *liked* being restrained by police and by security staff. I don't know the basis for this need; perhaps it made him feel safe. It could be that in his distorted view of relationships he saw being restrained as a gesture of care. Or perhaps there was a bondage aspect. But he often requested restraints or made them necessary by his erratic behaviour.

With all this in mind (it pays to read the patient's hospital chart *before* seeing the patient), I scanned the record of the current visit and saw that EMS had first taken Alan to the psychiatric hospital because he said he'd swallowed a large dose of Epival and had allegedly tried to cut off his surgically-created penis. Staff at the psychiatric facility had sent him to Sinai so that we could check first on his medical condition. The police had him mildly restrained in the waiting room, holding down his arms and legs as gently as they could.

Part of his ER routine was to create a massive scene and then refuse to have blood work done or co-operate with the examination.

"I want to be restrained!" he screamed.

"Before I can consider that I need you to answer my questions," I told him, knowing full well that he didn't have to tell me anything.

Alan would not let me take his blood pressure, so I was reduced to a cursory examination. We call that a "veterinary workup" because we base most of our findings on observation—something we imagine veterinarians do all the time. Although I wasn't able to determine his temperature, I could see he didn't look feverish or otherwise, which he likely would have been if in the midst of an overdose. Nor was he in any obvious physical pain, which a cut-up penis would almost certainly have evoked, not to mention a trail of blood. He wouldn't let me listen to his chest, but I observed that his pupils were clear and reactive to light, another indication he hadn't taken drugs, at least not excessively.

My next procedure was to ask him three questions to see if he was alert and oriented to person, place and time:

"What's your name?"

"I'm Alan. You fucking know my name. Why are you asking me that?"

"Do you know where you are?"

"I'm in fucking Sinai."

"Do you know what day it is?"

"It's fucking Saturday in the morning. What do you want?"

It was obvious by his responses that he was alert and oriented.

Once again I asked him to let me take a blood sample.

"Get the fuck away from me!" he screamed.

At this point I decided the show must no longer go on. I turned to the police, who were engrossed in the little drama being played out. "There's nothing wrong with him as far as I can see," I said. "He's discharged. Take him out."

"Do you want us to bring him back to the psychiatric hospital?" one of them asked.

"Just escort him off the premises," I said.

They looked at me in stunned confusion. It was not their business to know that we develop a specific and individual care plan for difficult patients such as Alan, or that I was implementing it at that moment. This was not what they had expected to be told to do. Alan also stared at me, but he was no longer screaming or swearing. There was a resigned look in his eyes that I felt was an acknowledgement that this round had gone to me. He had tried gamely but failed. The police did as I requested, albeit somewhat nervously, and ushered him out. He didn't come back that morning, and as far as I know he was fine. If something had happened to him I would have definitely been informed.

While Alan's routine often included very real assaults on his body, there are other patients, usually females, who have something called pseudo- (or fake) seizures. People with pseudoseizures usually have an underlying psychiatric problem in which attention seeking is a strong component. Unfortunately for those of us who work in the ER, they usually tie up a lot of resources.

There are several dramatic ways of getting attention in the emergency department. One is to stop breathing. Another is to faint and keel over. Taking off your clothes or urinating in the waiting room works quite nicely. So does having a seizure. A real seizure has to be attended to right away, in case the patient dies. That means a pseudoseizure has to be taken seriously until you know it's not real.

During a genuine seizure people rhythmically contract and relax their muscles in what's called a tonic-clonic, which is a tense, rhythmic contraction. These used to be called grand mal seizures, but that term has gone out of favour. Tonic-clonics are the contractions commonly associated with epilepsy. The patients often foam at the mouth, may pucker or smack their lips, and are unresponsive.

When someone is faking a seizure, she is actually awake and responsive. A quick and clever way to determine whether a patient is awake or not is called "cold water calorics." Using a syringe, you inject cold water into the patient's right ear and see how the eyes move in response. In patients who aren't faking, such as those with brain damage, the eyes will move toward the ear being irrigated. Patients with that kind of test response have a very poor prognosis. But if the patient is "awake and with the program," as we like to say, running cold water into the right ear will make the eyes begin jerking rhythmically back and forth quickly to the left and more slowly to the right. We call those jerky motions nystagmus.

Proving a patient is faking unconsciousness is the easy part. Often, you can say gently that you know the seizure isn't real. But some patients don't get the message. In these cases, you have to try a different approach.

The black art of stopping a pseudoseizure or telling the patient you know she is awake is to suggest rather loudly that you're going to do some procedure that is less than pleasant. One of my favourites is to threaten to intubate the patient. I say it right close to the patient's head: "This looks like a serious seizure and we're going to have to intubate the patient now." Then I will open up the laryngoscope blade and bring it to the tip of the tongue; that is the moment when the hand comes up to stop me.

I used another, even more effective, technique on a woman who was obviously a highly skilled faker. I wasn't aware of her past history of pseudoseizures and had tried giving her some Valium to stop the supposed seizure, but to no effect. By this point I began to sense she was not having a genuine episode. A colleague in neurology had recently suggested a surefire way to unmask a faker. It was time to try it out. I moved close to the patient and said to the nurses who were assisting me: "The medication doesn't seem to be working when we give it to her through the IV. We're going to have to give it to her in the eye." That did the trick. She immediately sat up. "I feel better," she said. "I can go home now." And she did.

Most experts discourage that kind of stuff, but when an ER is overcrowded and other sick and suffering people need our help, we can't waste time with methods that might work, given enough time to enact them. I admit that sometimes I've put people into four-point restraints—both arms and legs are tied down—and sedated them when verbal de-escalation might have worked. In verbal de-escalation, you have to weigh the risk that things will quickly get out of control. A volatile patient could take a hostage or throw furniture through a window and shatter the glass, which could cut other patients or staff. Sometimes you need rapid control. Sometimes it feels like you need a dart gun.

I was thinking of Alan and of the story Croskerry had told me as I finished my examination of Pat, the ranting patient. He never stopped his endless, incomprehensible monologue no matter what I said or did. It was not enjoyable being around him, and I had to exercise discipline to see him as a unique patient and not frame him as just another disturbed person. All his tests had come back and he had nothing medically wrong with him. The next step was to send him to the psychiatric hospital.

There is an ebb and flow of patients who appear to have mental health problems between the Mount Sinai ER and the psychiatric facility. Our role at the ER is to determine whether a patient needs to be seen by a psychiatrist and whether there's a medical cause for erratic behaviour—a person can seem to be suffering from a mental concern such as schizophrenia when, in fact, the behaviour is the result of a brain injury. Because of that possibility, the psychiatric hospital often sends someone who was first brought there (or who arrived voluntarily) over to the ER to be checked out medically, and the ER often sends someone who first arrived on our doorstep over to the psychiatric hospital if we find him to be medically fit but in need of psychiatric help. When the latter is the case, we send the patient to a nearby psychiatric facility to see a psychiatrist. In most cases, they go voluntarily. However, if we think they're suffering from a psychiatric condition, are a danger to themselves and/or to others, or if they appear not to be competent to look after themselves, we have to fill out a form before having the patient transferred to the centre. In our lingo we say a patient has been "formed." This is a reference to "Form 1" under the Ontario Mental Health Act, which allows us to detain and restrain for up to seventy-two hours patients that we suspect are suffering from a psychiatric illness and are either a danger to themselves or others or who lack the competence to care for themselves.

A Form 1 doesn't confer the right to hold a patient for longer than seventy-two hours, nor does it compel the patient to be treated. There's another psychiatric form dealing with compulsory treatment that the admitting psychiatrist may have to fill out if he or she wants to treat the patient's psychiatric condition against their will. There's another issue as well. If I want to order a blood test to check the patient's alcohol level and they refuse, I may have to honour that decision if the patient appears to be competent to refuse treatment, even though they have a psychiatric illness. Things can get really confusing.

Once we have "formed" someone, we can move him over to the psychiatric hospital. We only send adults there; we might refer a child or youth to Sick Kids, although it doesn't have a locked ward. If underage patients require confinement, we have to search for a facility that can handle them, which can eat up a lot of time.

I never found out what happened to Pat after he went to the psychiatric facility. That's typical in emergency medicine. Often we aren't told what happens to our patients after we refer them to other hospitals. It's possible he is now on a medication that makes life manageable for him and those around him. But I have my doubts that all is well in his life. He seemed to be in a deep psychotic hole. I see a lot of Pats in the ER—lost souls who are trapped in a world of delusion and paranoia. Few return to us in a healthy state. It's easy to dismiss them as "nut jobs." It takes discipline to see them as human beings, especially if you are sleep deprived and exhausted from trying to help an endless parade of people who seem to have "real" medical problems. They deserve the same care and concern as everyone else. I keep reminding myself of that. I don't ever want to stop caring. But sometimes, the more outrageously patients behave, the harder it is to keep that precept in mind.

CHAPTER FIVE

MOONLIGHTERS AND FREQUENT FLYERS

1:33 A.M.

My next patient had been waiting for more than three hours, which was not long considering her circumstances. If it had been a crazy night she could have been sitting tight a lot longer. Her stated reason for coming just happened to fall into an aspect of medicine that's a specialty of mine. My curiosity more than anything else made me intrigued to see her.

Elena was a stout woman in her early fifties. Her skin was the kind of bloodless white that suggested a lifetime of heavy smoking. Her husband, who looked considerably older, accompanied her. He was overweight, and he emitted a mild wheeze as he rose to greet me. His hands were covered in liver spots.

When I asked Elena to explain her situation she spun quite the story. She and her husband were flying to the United States later that morning for a lengthy visit. They lived in Moncton and had stopped over in Toronto for a few days. She was on the strong painkiller OxyContin for a chronic back problem and had been given a large prescription by her doctor before she left. Unfortunately, she had left her bottle of pills on the plane from Halifax. She called Air Canada as soon as she realized what had happened, but the bottle had not been turned in or found by the cleaning crew. As she told her tale her husband nodded at the appropriate moments, like a one-man Greek chorus.

It was an impressive yarn, and I gave her full credit for the detail, imagination and convenient circumstances. First of all, back pain isn't really a diagnosis, in that it doesn't tell me what's going on inside Elena's back. She might have had pain coming from arthritis in her spine, or from chronically strained muscles, a condition we call myofascial pain syndrome. She might have had pain that comes from inflamed or irritated nerves along the spine, what's known as neuropathic pain.

I can and sometimes do order a CT scan or an MRI of the back to try and diagnose the problem. Everybody, and I mean *everybody*, who comes in with back pain expects to get a CT or an MRI or at least some plain ordinary X-rays. What they don't realize is that in the vast majority of patients, CTs and MRIs fail to show the cause of chronic back pain. Oh sure, they might show me that Elena had arthritis in the spine. But so do I and several million people walking around North America.

A study published in 1994 in the *New England Journal of Medicine* found that 38 percent of test subjects who underwent MRIs had bulging discs in their spine, while 90 percent had degenerative disc disease of the spine, which is code in medicine for arthritis. Sounds scary. Here's the kicker: not one single person who participated in the study had any pain whatsoever in the spine. The study's authors concluded that, in most cases, "the discovery by MRI of bulges or protrusions in people with low back pain may be coincidental."

A study published in the *Journal of the American Medical Association* randomly assigned 380 patients with back pain to receive either MRIs or basic X-rays of the spine. The patients who underwent MRIs were no better off than those who got X-rays, although they did end up having more visits to the doctor and more treatments, and were more likely to have surgery. The findings of these and other studies have led organizations like the American Pain Society and the American College of Physicians to discourage doctors from ordering MRIs for people with chronic back pain.

Where does that leave me with a patient like Elena, who might scream, moan, cry, limp, and have all kinds of trouble getting on and off the examining table? She might be telling the truth, or she could be a complete and utter phony.

That's the conundrum about back and other forms of chronic pain. Despite amazing advances in medicine and diagnosis, pain is still a subjective complaint. If you say you have a fever, I can check your temperature. If you say your throat is sore, I can look for redness and pus on your tonsils. But I can't verify chronic pain. At the end of the day, I pretty well have to rely on what you tell me. Real back pain can be horrible. It can make every moment of the day unbearable. It might be so bad you have to go on long-term disability. I know of several patients who committed suicide because of blinding, unremitting body pain. I know this because for nearly ten years I had an office practice in which I saw patients with chronic pain. I've seen careers and marriages ruined, and lives destroyed.

In an ideal world, I could save myself a lot of time by simply writing Elena a script (prescription) for OxyContin to replace the supply she had allegedly lost.

But this is not an ideal world.

OxyContin is the brand name of a controlled-release form of

the powerful narcotic oxycodone, manufactured by Purdue Pharma. The FDA approved it in 1995 and Health Canada in 1996. In terms of efficacy, oxycodone is pretty much on a par with morphine, the most powerful narcotic pain reliever we have in our arsenal. Oxy-Contin was approved for chronic pain due to cancer as well as for chronic back and other causes of pain not associated with cancer. Other forms of oxycodone last for three to four hours. But Oxy-Contin's time-release formula means that a single dose of the drug lasts between eight and twelve hours for most patients, making it ideal for people who have constant, daily pain.

I have to make an important disclosure here. As I developed expertise in detecting prescription drug abuse and diversion, as well as in chronic pain management, I began to be asked to share my knowledge and experience with colleagues. Over the past twenty years, I've given hundreds of lectures and seminars to physicians, nurses, pharmacists and even law enforcement officers across Canada and around the world.

In the early 1990s, I began to be paid by a pharmaceutical company to lecture health professionals at hospital rounds or at continuing medical education events, such as conferences and dinner meetings. As well, I appeared in a number of educational videos on pain management and prescription drug abuse that were supported by educational grants from drug companies. If I travelled to another city to give the talk, it was on the company's dime. I was put up in five-star hotels and taken to nice restaurants. When I travelled across the continent, I was invariably given a ticket in business class.

To my knowledge, the companies that sponsored my talks had no direct input into the opinions I expressed. I'm not saying there weren't moments that crossed the line. I remember wrapping up a talk in Calgary when a very high-strung manager at a drug company took me aside and yelled at me for talking too positively about a competitor's product. But that manager is long gone from the company.

Occasionally, I gave talks paid for by other drug companies. I can remember being interviewed for a video sponsored by another pharmaceutical company. Top brass from the company showed up to watch the taping. Tape rolling, the interviewer asked me a question that I answered. The company guy didn't like my answer. The tape was stopped while the manager huddled with the interviewer, out of earshot. Discussion finished, the camera was turned back on and I was asked the question again. My answer was the same. He asked again, in a slightly different way. After five or six attempts to get me to rephrase my answer, I began to sound like a robot. This went on for an hour or so. Eventually, they stopped the interview. I promised myself I'd never do another interview for that company again.

Whenever my fee was paid by a drug company, there was full disclosure to that effect to conference attendees and organizers alike.

As I gave these talks, I convinced myself that I was able to educate thousands of health professionals and law enforcement officers. I also got the sense that the entire world of organized medicine was blasé about growing links between Big Pharma and continuing medical education. Major medical conferences were heavily sponsored by pharmaceutical companies; they're the ones with the huge exhibit halls where drug companies shill their wares to conference attendees. One conference organizer told me that without sponsorship from pharmaceutical companies, the cost of conference tuition would double, driving tens if not hundreds of physicians away.

Not everyone was comfortable with what Big Pharma was doing.

Joel Lexchin is a fellow emergency physician at University Health Network and also teaches at the School of Health Policy and Management at Toronto's York University. Lexchin has been an outspoken critic of the involvement of pharmaceutical sponsorship of continuing medical education. Alan Cassels is a drug policy researcher at the University of Victoria and co-author, with Ray Moynihan, of the 2005 book *Selling Sickness: How the World's Biggest Pharmaceutical Companies Are Turning Us All into Patients.*

In a letter to the *Canadian Medical Association Journal,* Lexchin and Cassels had this to say about the reasons why pharmaceutical companies pay for continuing medical education, known far and wide by the initials CME:

> The people who run pharmaceutical companies don't give gifts; rather, they make investments, on which they expect a return. In the case of CME, the total 'gift' in the United States is in the range of U.S.$700 million annually. Gifts such as direct or indirect financial assistance to attend CME are part of the culture of reciprocity so important in physician–industry relations, and such gifts can create unconscious obligations in physicians that industry knows will be repaid in one way or another.

In the years since I started giving talks sponsored by drug companies, a growing chorus of critics has condemned company-sponsored continuing medical education. In September 2008, Eli Lilly and Company announced that beginning in 2009, it would post online all its payments to doctors for speaking and consulting services. At the time, the company said the postings would "likely include" the names of the doctors, or would provide some other identifying information about them, along with the reason for the payment, according to the *New York Times.* In the wake of Eli Lilly's announcement, drug maker Merck & Company said it too would disclose speaking fees it pays to doctors. So far, Canadian pharmaceutical companies have not followed suit.

I had my office practice in chronic pain at the time OxyContin came on the market. For a good percentage of my patients, the drug was highly effective at reducing pain and helping them get on with their lives.

As prescription drugs go, OxyContin was a huge seller. By 2001 it was the best-selling non-generic narcotic pain reliever in the U.S. It was also extremely popular in Canada. As legal sales grew so too did its illegal use. Drug abusers quickly discovered that if OxyContin was crushed and smoked or injected intravenously, they experienced a powerful and immediate rush.

Often referred to on the street as "hillbilly heroin," OxyContin caused thousands of overdose deaths in the first decade of the century throughout North America, many of them in rural parts of the country. Both legitimate users and street users found that Oxy-Contin could quickly become habit forming. I sensed Elena was likely the former but I couldn't know for certain without checking out her story.

If a doctor wants to suss out the drug seeker as opposed to the legitimate patient, it helps to become a bit of a lie detector. I loved the way Elena said she had lost her prescription. I've had some patients tell me their bottle of narcotics was stolen from the glove box of their car. Others have told me they accidentally spilled an open bottle of pills into the toilet. You know what? It's always controlled substances like narcotics that get lost, stolen or dumped. It's never pills for blood pressure or diabetes.

Then there was the ticking clock. Many a good action thriller has a bomb that's counting down to detonation or a looming dead-line of some sort. Elena and her hubby had a plane to catch in a few hours. That explained why she had come to the ER. That put pressure on me to help her out without asking too many questions, if any at all. But thrillers also need plot twists and unexpected coincidences. That was my contribution. Elena had no idea how much I knew about prescription drug abuse.

I asked Elena for the name of her physician in New Brunswick and the pharmacy where she acquired her prescriptions. A flash of fear, like a jagged lightning bolt, lit up her eyes. She hesitated for a moment, parsing the pros and cons of answering. No fool, she quickly regrouped and provided the information. Her husband fidgeted. I said I would be back shortly.

I was convinced that Elena was a drug seeker who also fell under a broad category of people we frequently see at the ER called "moonlighters"—patients who flit from hospital to hospital in hope of convincing an ER physician to write them out a prescription. The scourge of ERs, they drop in to a hospital where they've never been before and that has no medical history of them on file, even travelling to different cities once they've made the rounds of all the ERs where they live.

One time a woman came to Mount Sinai asking for Demerol to relieve a terrible migraine. This is a favourite lament of moonlighters because a migraine, like back pain, is easy to fake and virtually impossible to prove. You either believe the person or you don't. A real migraine can be awful to endure, so there's a lot of pressure on the physician to err on the side of prescribing rather than denying pain medication. Unfortunately for the patient, I have an excellent memory for faces.

"I remember seeing you at another hospital I used to work at," I said. "Didn't you ask for Demerol then for a kidney problem?" I watched her face closely to see her reaction. She tried to mask her surprise.

"You must be mistaken," she said, clearly taken aback.

I smiled and said quietly: "I don't think so. Are you sure you need Demerol? How about some Advil?"

She muttered something I couldn't catch and bolted out of the ER. On other occasions I have asked moonlighters to tell me their family doctor's name and contact information. Even if it's late at night or early in the morning, I try to track the physician down to confirm the person needs the medication. Just knowing I'm going to do that makes some of them turn tail and leave. That was how I intended to check out Elena's story.

Moonlighters are not always making up an ailment. They can have a legitimate problem that requires pain medication. But those who have become addicted to the drug have gradually exceeded the amount their doctor prescribed. They might be looking at a week or longer before being able to obtain their next prescription legitimately. Again, I have gone to great efforts to contact the doctor, even if it means the person has to wait a long time at the ER. I don't do this to be difficult but to protect the patient from possible problems. Many of the drugs they take are powerful and can cause damage to the liver or other organs if overconsumed.

How desperate are some people for their fix? I've seen a patient agree to undergo a spinal tap, which can be a most painful procedure, to justify getting his meds.

During the 1980s I often lectured on what I saw as the folly of prescribing pain medication too liberally. I harped on the scams I'd seen—by this point I was very good at detecting scammers and had developed a reputation as an international expert from my considerable writing and presentations on the subject—and offered tips to physicians on how to suss out drug seekers.

At some point in the late 1980s I became aware of a recurring response to my talks. Quite a few medical professionals came up to me after a presentation and suggested I could be doing some harm. A typical comment was that I was putting out a message that when a patient asked for pain relief our response should be to "just say no."

I remember one confrontation with a woman who was quite intense. "What if someone is screaming in pain after having received two injections but the staff ignore her?" she said, pointing a finger at me accusingly. "They're not very sympathetic, because you've convinced them the person is faking."

I began to wonder if perhaps she and the others who made the same observation might be right. For one thing, I knew that nurses, who are often the ones who can best communicate a patient's needs to the doctors, tended to be conservative when it came to doling out pain medication. If you instruct nurses to administer pain meds in a range of fifty to seventy-five milligrams they will often choose fifty. If you tell them to give a patient a drug every four to six hours they will choose six, which often becomes longer depending on what else they have to deal with. By that time the previous dosage may have worn off.

By the end of the 1980s, I was seriously rethinking my philosophy toward pain medication. In 1990 that evolution culminated in a documentary I prepared for the CBC Radio series *Ideas* called "The Politics of Pain," in which I explored "the medical profession's inability to treat chronic pain effectively and compassionately," as the program's blurb proclaimed. This was a 180-degree turn for me. Dr. No had suddenly become Dr. Yes when it came to doling out pain-relieving meds.

Never one to step halfway onto a new street, I decided to put my new philosophy into action. I opened a chronic pain management practice, in addition to my work at the ER, and ran it for the next nine years. Not many doctors are willing to devote a considerable portion of their practice to this kind of work. It takes a large amount of time because it's not that easy to find the right pain medication for a patient. It's not uncommon to experiment with large and differing amounts of drug cocktails over several years. You change the dosage, switch narcotics, monitor side effects, manage a patient's tolerance levels for the drugs, and so on. It requires constant research into the new drugs available on the market and any problems that arise with existing ones. It's also emotionally draining, as you're constantly dealing with people suffering varying degrees of debilitating pain, people who are often at the end of their rope.

One of my first patients was a woman who had suffered a stroke. As a result she had nerve pain that was so searing she walked around all day clutching her face. By this time I knew my role was to do whatever I could to alleviate her suffering, no matter how many drugs I gave her. If managing chronic pain was financially lucrative, more practitioners might be enticed to the field, but it's not. Quite the opposite. It generates low billings and, therefore, low pay.

As I embraced my new approach I went from worrying about drug scammers to being one of the first physicians in Canada to prescribe large doses of narcotics to people in pain. I also came to the awareness that those of us in the ER world managed pain poorly, that we tended to undertreat it. The underlying reason, I believed, was a kind of "narcophobia." We assumed, as a profession, that if we gave patients a lot of narcotics they'd become addicted.

Always thirsty for information, I began taking courses in the U.S., where the attitude toward pain management seemed to be more progressive. I was particularly inspired by a presentation by two leading ER doctors—Paul Paris and Ronald Stewart (the one and the same Doc Hollywood we met earlier in the book). In 1987 they published the textbook *Pain Management in Emergency Medicine,* which was a practical primer that demystified the issues I was becoming increasingly fascinated by.

Their course greatly influenced me. I discovered that in Canada we were in the Stone Age when it comes to understanding pain management. They introduced me to the dangers associated with

Demerol. If we did continue to administer it, they said, at least give it intravenously rather than as an intramuscular injection in the butt or the stomach, which can take much longer to provide relief. An IV injection absorbs into the bloodstream quickly and tends to reduce the need for repeated doses.

I returned to Toronto a convert to administering drugs through an IV, a radical concept at the time. The first time I asked a nurse to do this she looked at me as if I were crazy. She thought it would be too powerful and would stop a patient's breathing and could kill him. I assured her that wouldn't be the outcome, which, of course, it wasn't. I urged my colleagues to accept this new and better method and eventually convinced them. Change did come, but slowly at times. When we began using IVs to deliver narcotics it wasn't uncommon for a surgical resident, if brought in, say, for someone with severe abdominal pain, to write on the patient's chart in large letters: "I cannot properly assess this patient because he received a narcotic. He's nodding off. And the drug will mask his symptoms." It took authoritative studies showing this to be untrue to put this attitude to rest.

I was becoming a bit of a radical, although I didn't see myself that way at the time. I just knew a voice inside me was beginning to challenge how we functioned as doctors, especially when it came to being truthful with ourselves and our patients about how the profession really worked.

An example of just how much my philosophy had changed occurred in 1990 when I began treating Sally, a middle-aged woman who had been badly injured in three car accidents, each one compounding the pain imposed by the previous one. Sally suffered from what's known as failed back syndrome, which refers to pain in the back and legs that develops after spinal surgery. She had run out of surgical options by the time she ended up in my office and was left with the prospect of debilitating pain for the rest of her life. For her, pain relief was the only sliver of light in what had become a horrible existence.

I started her out on as high a dosage of morphine as I thought she could handle and slowly, over a period of almost two years, inched her up to where she was taking 4,000 milligrams a day. Several hundred milligrams a day is a common dosage. The amount I gave her could kill someone who hadn't been carefully eased into such an intense regimen. For Sally, it made life manageable. On 4,000 milligrams a day she could function and was even able to drive a car, which was impossible when she first came to see me.

The last few years have seen major changes in the profession's approach to pain management. The emphasis has definitely shifted toward developing and prescribing drugs that make pain as bearable as possible. Unfortunately, that liberalized approach to pain management has led in a growing number of instances to doctors being too willing to prescribe narcotics when they aren't necessary.

We have lots of data on the scale of the problem of prescription drug abuse in the United States. There's not been much research done on this problem in Canada, however. That will change with a study commissioned in 2009 by the Canadian Institute for Health Research, a federal government funding body. Under the leadership of Benedikt Fischer, PhD, a team, of which I'm a member, will try to determine, among other findings, how many people are acquiring OxyContin and similar drugs from doctors, and the degree to which it has become a recreational rather than medicinal pill. We will also be researching the number of deaths attributed to prescription drug overdoses, and what role, if any, other stimulants and depressants, such as Valium and alcohol, play in them. At the moment such information is not being gathered, so we don't know, for example, if someone who dies from an OxyContin overdose obtained the drugs legitimately or on the street. It should prove to be a fascinating and invaluable project.

Though I couldn't be sure, my gut told me Elena was using OxyContin herself as opposed to selling it to drug dealers. I telephoned her pharmacy, which fortunately was open twenty-four hours a day, and identified myself. For security reasons they had to call me back through the Mount Sinai switchboard, which they did right away. I would have contacted her doctor, but I didn't see the need to have his answering service wake him up unless the pharmacy refused to help. The pharmacist confirmed that Elena had recently filled an eight-week prescription for OxyContin, although it was three weeks earlier than the date she had told me. He also noted the daily dosage set by her doctor.

"One of the reasons I was so willing to speak with you," the pharmacist added, "was when you mentioned you were calling about a prescription for Elena. We are very familiar with her. She has a record of overusing her medication and seeking refills from other doctors and clinics. She's what we call—"

"—a moonlighter," I said, finishing the pharmacist's sentence.

"Yes, indeed. She's a moonlighter. She has a signed contract with her doctor that sets out how many pills she will get from him over a specific period of time. Plus she has agreed not to seek medication from any other physician other than her doctor or one of his partners at the clinic they all work at."

Armed with this information I returned to Elena and her husband. When I revealed what I had found out, she almost folded her body in disappointment.

"By my calculation," I said, "you should have five weeks' worth of pills left. That's enough for your trip."

She began to panic and reiterated that her pills had been left on the plane. "I can call Air Canada tomorrow and ask for a copy of the report you filed," I said, never intending to do such a thing. She gave up on that tactic and tried another approach.

"Okay, I used them up too quickly, but I was going through a really hard time," she said. I sympathized. This woman was clearly addicted and I knew OxyContin withdrawal was no fun. But I had to remind her that the agreement she made with her doctor tied my hands.

"Oh, but I didn't think that agreement was valid in Ontario," she said, her husband softly echoing this last desperate point. I almost burst out laughing. I then told her to cancel her trip to the U.S., wondering to myself if indeed it was ever a reality, and go back home. "You need help to deal with your dependency. It's only going to get worse if you don't."

The couple gathered up their things and left. My guess was they would head for another ER and try their luck there. If I had to bet, I'd wager they would eventually succeed and acquire a new prescription. Elena's story was believable and as the night wore on and my colleagues at the other ERs became worn down with fatigue, she'd find someone who would not bother to conduct due diligence, as I had, and would just fill out a script. Unfortunately, I couldn't warn nearby ERs, as doing so would violate Elena's privacy and might compromise her ability to receive appropriate care.

I have lectured far and wide on the problem of prescription drug abuse and diversion. As I've shown you, I warned that Oxy-Contin abuse in Canada was likely to occur. As the abuse of this drug began to be reported here, I strengthened my admonitions to health professionals who attended my talks to be careful prescribing Oxy-Contin to patients, and to watch for signs of abuse and diversion. However, in light of what's happened, I have to ask myself whether my involvement with pharmaceutical companies strengthened those warnings or blunted them. I also wonder whether speaking at events

sponsored by drug companies sent an unconscious signal to physicians that the problem of OxyContin abuse must be manageable, or
I wouldn't have agreed to having my talks sponsored.

I don't know the answers to those questions. But I do know
that they're always on my mind whenever I see patients like Elena.

2:04 A.M.

The encounter with Elena had eaten up almost thirty minutes. I
walked quickly through the ward, as I always do, to find my resident
and catch up on what she had been doing. Up ahead I saw a familiar
patient strapped onto a hallway gurney with four-point restraints. It
was Buddy, a sometimes-homeless guy who ended up in the ER far
too often for our liking. I could see some scraped skin on Buddy's
face, the result no doubt of a dust-up on the street or in a bar. We
had become convinced over time that Buddy picked fights that he
either knew he'd lose, or that he lost deliberately, so he could be
brought in for treatment. Fortunately he had never been badly beat-
en up, but he was playing a form of Russian roulette. It was only a
matter of time before one of his encounters caused him really serious
damage or possibly killed him. Buddy was what we call a "frequent
flyer," a patient who repeatedly checks in to the ER.

There are many reasons why the frequent flyers come to us.
Some want a warm place to sleep. Or they need to be comforted,
to have someone care for them. The bleeding heart in me says that
most of them have no other place to go for medical services. In
2008, Statistics Canada estimated as many as 4.1 million Canadians
didn't have a family physician. When these patients need to be seen,
they go to walk-in clinics, urgent care centres and emergency departments. The emergency chart that is cranked out for every arriving

patient has a box in which the admitting clerk enters the name of the patient's family physician. Many of the patients we see these days have the initials NFD (No Family Doctor) inscribed in that box.

Family physicians have a name for people who don't have a family doc. They call them "orphan patients." A patient doesn't start out life legally attached to a physician, the way a child does to a parent. You can sign up with any physician you wish, provided the doctor accepts you into his or her practice. And unlike the relationship you have with your parents, when your family physician retires, moves away, dies, or kicks you out of the practice, you're free to seek out any MD (or, increasingly, any nurse practitioner) willing to look after you.

To me, the label "orphan patient" has a Dickensian feel to it, reminiscent of the government-run poorhouses of Victorian times that gave shelter to the destitute. Having adopted two children from orphanages in Russia, my heart aches for the prepubescent resident of an orphanage who is scrubbed clean and dressed up in the unlikely hope of being picked by prospective parents.

Orphan patients are a lot like that. They tend to have baggage that makes them unattractive even to young family physicians who are just starting out and have yet to fill their practice. Blame it on the system of paying family physicians for taking care of us. According to the 2007 National Physician Survey, roughly half of Canada's family physicians received more than 90 percent of their income from what is called "fee-for-service." That's a polite term for piecework; family physicians on fee-for-service receive a government-negotiated flat fee for every service performed. Depending on the province, that fee is often on the order of $25 to $35 per visit. After the family doctor deducts 30 to 50 percent of that fee to pay for office overhead, it's not a lot of money.

As a result, family physicians on fee-for-service often feel a sense of time pressure to see and treat each patient quickly and move on to the next. Paul Freedman, a veteran family physician in Toronto with nearly forty years' experience, teaches family practice residents at the Granovsky Gluskin Family Medicine Centre at Mount Sinai Hospital. He knows the daily grind of making a living as a fee-for-service family physician only too well.

"I'm doing ten times as much now with complex patients," he said on *White Coat, Black Art.* "Never mind the eighty-five-year-old who's got diabetes, congestive heart failure, chronic renal failure, dermatitis, bones that don't work, a head that's getting forgetful, and a pack load of pills that you have to sort out each time and care-givers you have to speak to." How many patients an hour would he like to see, to make a financial go of it? "If I could get away with four patients an hour or five patients an hour, life would be good. Some days it's like eight patients in an hour or some ridiculous amount like that. You feel like you're on a treadmill. I'm used to it, but it burns young kids out. They get trapped on this treadmill, and if they start to slow down significantly, the overhead eats them for breakfast."

At four patients an hour, the physician has an average of fifteen minutes to spend with each person, including the time it takes to write up notes about the visit in the patient's chart. At six patients an hour, we're talking ten minutes a patient. If the person brings up a second or a third problem, starts crying about a family issue, or even takes a few moments extra to get on and off the examining table, the physician can slip far behind schedule very quickly.

With that kind of time crunch, it's not surprising young family physicians who are building up a practice cherry-pick the easier "low-maintenance" patients. These days, family physicians like Dr. Omer Chaudhary of Strathroy, a town west of London, Ontario, are very careful about screening out prospective patients who they figure will take too much time. Chaudhary learned the process of screening patients systematically during his residency in family medicine. He first asks all prospective patients to fill out an application form. If he likes what he sees on the form, he invites the patient in for what family docs call a "meet and greet," a session that sounds a lot like a job interview.

"You have a group of patients out there who are doctor shoppers and who are drug seekers," he said on *White Coat, Black Art*. "As a medical student, you are forewarned about these patients. The application process allows me to get a sense of patients who I think may fall into that category. The other issue is that I want to develop a practice with only a certain proportion of elderly patients, maybe about 30 to 40 percent. For me, as a new family doctor, I find it difficult, when you have a patient with a long medical history and several medical problems, to see a respectable number of patients per day. If I can see a good thirty to forty people a day, I think that's my goal. If I have a lot of people where I have trouble juggling their problems and seeing them in a respectable timeline, I don't think I can meet that goal."

The patients who tend to get cherry-picked are the younger ones and those with few, if any, chronic medical problems. Those most likely to get passed over include seniors, especially those with complex medical problems, as well as patients with dementia, disabilities, chronic pain, alcohol and drug abuse, and psychiatric problems.

Sometimes, depending on where they live, even young and healthy patients have trouble finding a family doctor. It's estimated that between 20,000 and 30,000 orphan patients live in Sudbury, Ontario. In November 2008, Christina Clark attended a walk-in clinic in Sudbury, where she got a blood test that confirmed she was pregnant. The physician who saw Clark advised her to find herself a family physician. "I hadn't had a family physician for a year and a half," she told me on *White Coat, Black Art*. "I went on the website of the College of Physicians and Surgeons for the Greater City of Sudbury, and I called 126 [doctors] and I got 'no' every time."

Not surprisingly, many of the patients who don't get cherry-picked or who can't find a family doctor end up in the ER. It's frustrating because in many cases these patients are coming to us for routine family medicine care. When you're an adrenaline junkie like me, you prefer to rescue drowning patients, shock hearts that have stopped, and reset dislocated shoulders.

Moreover, unlike family practitioners, emergency physicians and nurses expect to see patients only once. Any time we see patients repeatedly, there's an almost instinctive letdown as soon as they arrive. "You again," I sometimes hear the triage nurse saying, echoing what most of us think. To ER doctors and nurses, repeat business means one of two things: we missed the diagnosis the first time (believe me, that happens all too often), or the patient is taking advantage of us because he has no other place to go and knows we can't refuse to treat him. At the same time, it can also mean that our discharge advice was confusing, that a follow-up appointment couldn't be arranged, or that a patient got a rash from the medication we prescribed. You learn to say "you again" at your peril.

———————

Before I took a quick look at Buddy, I automatically washed my hands with an alcohol sanitizer. The ER has dispensers every few feet apart, and they have become an essential part of our battle against the spread of hospital-bred diseases. Superbugs such as MRSA (Methicillin-resistant *Staphylococcus aureus*), VRE (Vanco-mycin-resistant *enterococcus*) and *Clostridium difficile,* better known as *C. difficile,* are the lead villains. It's not necessary for me to give a biology lesson on these nasty bugs; suffice it to say you don't want them in or on your body.

Each year nearly 250,000 Canadians get a hospital-acquired infection and about 12,000 die as a result. Here's the galling thing: half these deaths are preventable. Constant hand washing is the number one way to reduce what has become one of the leading causes of death in Canada.

The ubiquitous dispensers are, unfortunately, also a contributing factor to another type of frequent flyer. There is a small group of alcohol-dependent people (I am reluctant to use the term "alcoholic," which carries a slew of moral implications) who show up at the ER fairly often. Some come by ambulance, others just walk in and try to get admitted. It's not uncommon for them to have suffered a head injury from a fall or a fight, so it's important we examine them. When they're comatose from drinking, however, that's hard to do until they sober up enough for staff to take a medical history. The smart ones know this and sometimes pretend to be out cold when they're not. They're hoping we will place them on a gurney, usually in a hallway as the rooms are needed for people with more serious ailments. Their plan is to wait until they think no one is watching and steal some hand sanitizer, which they consume to become intoxicated.

Hand sanitizers contain up to 75 percent ethyl alcohol (a level necessary to kill microbes). Stealing hand sanitizer has become such a chronic problem that if I suspect a patient might be prone to this, I have him (it's usually a male) kept in the waiting room until I can conduct an examination. Despite our best efforts, a lot of patients succeed in their attempts and manage to down large quantities of sanitizer, which is not a safe thing to do. The primary reason is the danger of alcohol poisoning, of course, but there are other chemicals in the product, in smaller quantities, that could cause an allergic reaction.

While patients with alcohol dependency need to be watched closely around sanitizer, we also have to be careful that little children don't accidentally ingest it. A small dose can make a child quite ill. In 2007, a four-year-old girl in Tulsa, Oklahoma, was rushed to hospital after licking some hand sanitizer in her kindergarten class. She was found to have a blood alcohol reading of .085, which is high for an adult, never mind a child. Little children are often scampering around an ER department if they've come in with an ailing adult or their family and friends. They see adults using the sanitizer so it's natural to imitate our behaviour. Fortunately, I have not witnessed any children who have ingested sanitizer, but the American Association of Poison Control Centers' combined data from 2005 and 2006 found that poison control centres reported more than 20,000 exposures to hand sanitizer, with more than 17,000 cases involving children under the age of six.

All of us in the ER were aware that Buddy would drink the sanitizer if he had a chance. True, at the moment he was unresponsive to my questions and appeared to be sleeping off a bender, but I had learned that his acting skills were quite impressive.

A while later, I headed to the small kitchen area where all of us stash our food, anything from doughnuts—I know, some example we set—to plates of fruit. On the way back, I had to walk past Buddy. He was starting to stir.

"How're you doing?" I asked.

"I'm a little dry, doc," he said. "If you could let me out of these straps, I could get some water from the fountain."

I was certain his eye flickered toward the hand sanitizer dispenser for just a moment.

"I'll have the nurse bring you something," I said. "But nice try."

"Thanks, doc," he said. "I don't really like that stuff anyway," meaning the handwash. It was a transparent lie.

"Too salty?" I asked. "Not salty enough?"

"What are you talking about? You drunk?"

"Punch drunk, maybe," I said. "Must be the time of night."

Buddy laughed and settled back down on the gurney. I went off to have my snack. A couple of Timbits were left in a box by the sink. A sugar fix. Perfect. Just what I needed.

CHAPTER SIX

RESIDENTS AND LEASHES LONG AND SHORT

2:15 A.M.

The resident wanted me to see a suicidal woman who had arrived about midnight. At first it seemed like a straightforward case. It soon became anything but. In a way the woman was a repeat customer, but not because she was a frequent flyer. This was a troubled woman who had been at Mount Sinai after a botched suicide attempt.

The resident told me that Jessie was a recent immigrant from Scotland in her late forties. She had come to Toronto with her husband, who had accepted a promotion and job transfer with his international professional firm. Although they were now much better off financially, Jessie was homesick, her husband said, and had been pressuring him to quit and go back home. He told my resident this was not an option, as far as he was concerned. His wife, he added, "needed to accept her situation and honour her commitment to him and their marriage." The resident had found him to be stubborn and not very sympathetic to his wife's lot.

Her first suicide attempt had taken place about a week earlier. Jessie had been brought in by paramedics after swallowing a few pills of lorazepam and clomipramine. Lorazepam (Ativan) is used to calm anxiety and nerves. We often administer it in the ER to quiet agitated patients. It's a safe drug and works like Valium. Clomipramine, which was sold as Anafranil, is an old-style antidepressant that's often used to treat panic attacks and obsessive-compulsive disorder. It's rarely prescribed these days because it's potentially lethal if you take an overdose.

"How many pills of each did she swallow in her first suicide attempt?" I asked the resident.

"Her chart says she admits to having taken about five or six pills of each," she said.

A suicide gesture, I thought. Enough to get attention but not enough to die.

"What happened this time?"

"Her husband said she told him it was about forty Tylenol," the resident said. "I don't think he believed her. He seemed to think she made it up to get attention."

"What else do we know?"

"He says she has a drinking problem. She was slurring her words and seemed a bit drunk. Her husband says she has panic attacks, like really intense terror, afraid to go out of the house kind of thing. And he says she's really depressed."

"What's she on?"

"Gabapentin. That's, um, for . . ."

"Often for epilepsy," I said. This was a teaching moment. There's a large list of drugs to learn about and the best way for a resident to increase her knowledge is during a case history. "Also used as a mood stabilizer. People who are bipolar or manic-depressive are put on it to help balance them out. Seems appropriate based on what we know about her."

I told the resident to order blood work for Jessie, but she had already done that. Excellent initiative.

Then I asked one more question. "Anything that doesn't make sense to you?"

I have found over the years that this question, whether posed to a resident, to a colleague or to me, can elicit vital information, the kind that can sometimes take us from what seems to be one type of problem and make us explore, and eventually discover, other ones.

After a few moments my resident answered: "She's complaining of having a claw hand," she answered, "but she doesn't know why it's happening."

From the look on the resident's face, neither did she. I was busy with my own patients, but I decided I'd better see Jessie for myself.

Resident is short for *resident physician*. A resident is a recently graduated physician (that's right, they can rightfully call themselves doctors) who is doing postgraduate training in hospital. The length of postgraduate training depends on the program, and ranges from two years for a family physician to as long as six years for neurosurgery. On top of that, some physicians take extra training in the form of a fellowship. For instance, after completing a residency in orthopedics, a physician might do extra training to become a subspecialist in cancers that affect the bone.

They're called residents because up until three or four generations ago they used to *reside* at the hospital. In the United Kingdom, residents are called registrars. Here in Canada, I've heard them referred to as house officers, and again you can see the subtle reference to living and not just working inside the sliding doors. The only other grown-ups I can think of who do that are soldiers and prisoners.

There is a symbiotic relationship between residents and staff physicians like me. I teach them clinical medicine by letting them practise on my patients. In return, they see patients and lighten some of my workload. As a staff physician, I'm responsible for every patient my resident sees. Still, a bright resident who combines excellent book learning with good judgment takes care of my patients so well I hardly need to see them myself. The resident who is marginally competent slows me down by forcing me to double-check all of his or her findings. Occasionally, there are devious residents who lie when you ask them if they've done a physical examination or ordered a blood test. Fortunately, we see few of them.

Nowadays, residents do one- or two-month rotations through the ER. Often, it's not clear whether you can trust a resident's judgment until something bad happens to a patient. Once at the tail end of a night shift, many years ago, a colleague who works at a hospital in another province told me about a resident who spoke to him briefly during a shift about a patient with a red eye. The two discussed the possible causes, and they agreed that the resident would refer the patient to an ophthalmologist. When I say they had a brief conversation, I mean my colleague and the resident had a ten- or twenty-second chat in the hallway. Not nearly a long enough chat, it turned out. A few days later, the ophthalmologist rightfully reamed my colleague out for prescribing the patient corticosteroid eye drops, which is generally discouraged in emergency medicine because the complications can be serious and because the dosage needs to be carefully regulated. Fortunately, the ophthalmologist was able to fix things before the patient suffered any harm.

What was downright scary was that the resident said she'd told my colleague about her management plan and that he had agreed with it. Was this a slip-up on my colleague's part? Of course it could be. However, he said he didn't feel comfortable giving corticosteroid eye drops, and has rarely if ever done so on his own.

Bottom line is that ER docs have to keep residents on a leash. How long should the leash be? To answer that question, emergency physicians learn to assess residents quickly.

"I can usually size up residents within one shift or even a half shift," my ER colleague John Ross told me on *White Coat, Black Art*. "Can they speak with confidence, and do they have a good knowledge base, or are they one of those somewhat manipulative fakers? It's part of the eye contact, the body language, all of which tells me this guy knows what he's talking about, or this person doesn't know what they're talking about, and they're BS-ing me.

"Say the resident is telling me about a patient with chest pain," he continues. "I ask whether the patient smokes cigarettes, because I notice they didn't mention it when they were telling me the patient's history. If they pause for just a few nanoseconds before answering me, I know they didn't ask the patient. If after the pause, the resident says, 'No, they don't smoke,' I know the resident is lying. Those are the things that really annoy me. They should have asked, and now they're telling tales that may or may not be true."

Compounding the difficulty in deciding whether or not to trust a resident is the time pressure inherent in the ER.

"The phone is ringing," says Ross. "The nurse over there wants to talk to me. There's another medical student who has another patient to discuss with me. And I'm at the end of my shift, and I'm getting kind of tired. My wife wants me to be home. All of those sorts of issues play into the decision to go back and retake a history that a less-than-competent resident has just presented to me."

Meanwhile, just as we're sizing up the residents, they're doing the same to us. They test us to see if we know what we're talking about. Residents expect us to have up-to-date knowledge on every topic in emergency medicine. I often get the feeling I'm supposed to be a kind of jukebox of medical knowledge.

If a patient comes in with a suspected blood clot on the lungs or pulmonary embolus, they expect I should be able to deliver a perfect, evidence-based, two-minute mini-lecture on the various X-rays and blood tests used in the diagnosis. Suspected methanol poisoning? I'd better have a mini-talk on the pros and cons of fomepizole versus ethanol in the treatment.

If I were a surgeon, or a neurologist, or a gynecologist, the size of my medical jukebox would be limited. You don't ask an endocrinologist how to manage a brain tumour. But in emergency medicine, I'm expected to know a bit about everything. Trouble is, with the evolution of emergency medicine as a *serious* specialty, our mentors and many of my colleagues have bought into the notion that we're supposed to know a lot about every patient and every condition that walks through the ER doors.

When I was just out of residency myself, and the knowledge was fresh in my head, I could answer most of the residents' questions. Since then, medical knowledge has doubled more than once. But my brain hasn't. I live in fear of those moments when a resident asks me a question that I can't answer. Worse, I'm terrorized by the thought that a resident thinks I'm just a dumb old ER doc who is past his prime.

Who cares, you might ask? I do, and so do most of my colleagues. You see, residents may be down a notch in the power relationship with us attending doctors. But they've got one weapon and they know how to use it.

It's called the evaluation. Every month that a resident rotates

THE NIGHT SHIFT   111

through the ER, surgical or any other ward, they evaluate us (just as we evaluate them). And these days, resident evaluations wield a great deal of influence. If one resident disses the ER, no one pays too much attention. But if several start complaining about the hours, or the educational experience, or the teaching abilities of attendings like me. I've seen it turn into a full-blown crisis, with consequences for us and for the hospital.

Chronically bad evaluations from residents inevitably result in some sort of investigation, often by an independent third party. The consequences may include having residency positions cut from the hospital. If you're an attending and you depend on having residents help you see patients, losing them can be a disaster.

Therefore, ER doctors have to keep an eye on residents just as they keep an eye on us. It's easier for emergency physicians to keep tabs, because our job calls for us to be present at all times during our assigned shifts. It's a different story altogether for attending physicians and surgeons on other services. They do not spend all or even much of their working days with residents. To keep tabs on the patients admitted to their service, they make rounds with the residents once a day, or perhaps as little as two times a week. That means they're hopelessly dependent on residents being their eyes and ears on the wards.

———————————

The resident and I went to see Jessie in her room. She was disoriented and confused and slurring her words. She knew she was in a hospital but she wasn't able to tell me which one, nor did she know the month or the day. I checked her eyes and pupils, which both seemed normal. She was using her lips properly, and her neck was okay. Her vital signs were normal, although her heart rate was slightly elevated, but that often happens when someone is anxious. I sensed something was wrong with her beyond what we had been told. Her confusion should not have been caused by a Tylenol over-dose, if indeed she had ingested the number her husband had re-ported. What the hell do I do, I wondered?

With a patient who is confused, the book says wait until she wakes up and is less confused. See what pops up, if anything, from the blood work. And get a urine toxicology test done to see what, if anything, she has ingested. Unfortunately, Mount Sinai's lab was not capable of detecting Gabapentin. For that we had to use another facility, and the results could take a while. Our lab, however, could tell me if she had indeed gobbled down a massive number of Tylenol pills. If Jessie did have forty pills in her system, she wouldn't die immediately. She would develop a bit of nausea from the initial ingestion, but as it slowly became absorbed in her system, say over three or four days, it would poison her liver and she could die from liver failure.

The good news for Jessie was that a Tylenol overdose could be easily treated with another drug that has proven to be an antidote. In the old days we would have pumped her stomach. A flexible gavage tube, which looks like a slender garden hose, was inserted through the mouth into the throat, and from there eased into the stomach. A saline solution was then pumped into the stomach, which helped to suction out the contents.

This happened to me when I was six or seven years old. A curi-ous child, I had swallowed a handful of baby aspirin tablets. My parents rushed me to the closest ER. I will never forget that day. First they took my history. Then they came at me with what looked to a six-year-old like a tube of toothpaste. They squeezed out some gooey muck and shoved it in my mouth. Next came the tube. It felt as if I was being tortured. I can still remember the terrifying pumping sensation and the taste of salt in my throat. Trust me, I never swallowed anything I shouldn't have after that.

The problem with this approach was that it didn't always work. Unless someone had ingested a massive amount of drugs or some other unwanted substance that would take forever to pass into the body's system, the pumping came too late. The drugs were already moving through the liver and intestines.

Another method we sometimes employ is to give the person a bottle of activated charcoal with Sorbitol. The combo soaks up the poison and pushes it out the other end in one disgusting, tarry sludge. This little cocktail is not very pleasant to swallow.

Often, we would use both methods at once. We'd lubricate a nasogastric tube with some local anaesthetic and stick it into a nostril. The rule was to always check for a deviated septum because that nostril would be harder to manoeuvre the tube past. Threading the tube into the back of the throat was tricky, a trial-and-error process of searching for the right angle that was akin to safecracking. Once the tube was in place the patient was given a glass of water and asked to *swallow, swallow, swallow.* That helped the tube make it into the stomach. You knew it was there by injecting air through the tube and listening for a gurgling sound. The final act was to take a syringe filled with the activated charcoal/Sorbitol combo and send it down into the stomach through the tube. Oh, there was one more thing to do—get the hell out of the way as fast as possible. At least five or six times out of ten the patient would hurl black stuff all over the room. That is one of the reasons we don't use this method anymore. Another is that it never proved to be that successful.

Needless to say, I don't miss the nasogastric tube, and I'm just as happy when I don't have to use activated charcoal. For people who take an overdose of Tylenol, we give a lovely little drug called

Mucomyst that acts as an antidote to Tylenol poisoning. Muco-myst, or N-acetyl-cysteine, its generic name, was developed to help people with cystic fibrosis breathe better. But it was also found to have another benefit. It rejuvenates the liver by beefing up its ability to detoxify and get rid of acetaminophen, which is Tylenol. If Jessie indeed had a massive number of Tylenol in her system, we'd give her Mucomyst intravenously over a period of several hours. No tubes, no mess. Ain't progress grand?

I was still with Jessie when a nurse came in with the blood work results. Jessie's acetaminophen level was very high. Problem was, we didn't know how much Tylenol she had taken and when. It might have been about four hours earlier but there was no way to nail down the time for certain. That information was critical, since an elevated acetaminophen level is only diagnostic if taken between four and twenty-four hours following the overdose. A blood level taken less than four hours following ingestion is considered mean-ingless—even if it's elevated—because the result could be mislead-ing. There was also the nagging issue of her husband's implication that her story was fabricated. I looked at him and saw a deep fatigue in his face. Not just from the early morning hour, I thought. Also from having spent too much time in ER wards recently.

As I scanned Jessie's lab results, I saw something that altered the diagnosis and once again reminded me we should never frame a patient until we have all the facts. It was something the resident had missed completely. In addition to having a small amount of alcohol and several of her prescription drugs in her system, she had extremely low sodium (salt) levels. The normal range for an adult is between 135 and 145. Her level was 115, which was dangerously low.

This was life threatening. I've seen people die of seizures caused by low sodium. As soon as a person's sodium level is below 120, she suffers confusion, delirium, and possibly coma. Now things were starting to make sense. If Jessie was confused, the most likely cause was low sodium, not a drug overdose. It was even possible that she was suffering from a delusion she had overdosed on Tylenol, a delusion caused by low sodium rather than emotional problems. True, she had depression and had tried to commit suicide before; it's possible the low sodium level made her emotional issues worse.

Further tests revealed that her kidneys were not working well. When your sodium level is low the kidneys conserve sodium. Her kidneys weren't doing what they were supposed to. We call that SIADH, which stands for Syndrome Inappropriate ADH secretion. ADH stands for antidiuretic hormone, meaning she was spilling too much sodium in her urine when peeing.

The solution was to admit Jessie to hospital, where they put her on an IV drip of highly concentrated (hypertonic) saline. She soon bounced back and was her normal self in a few days. When I told her husband that there might be an organic and not a psychological cause for Jessie's erratic behaviour, he smiled a little but didn't seem to celebrate the news. I don't think he quite believed me. "Let's hope things change and she no longer wants us to go back to Glasgow," he said, a tired sadness in his voice. "It should make things better," I said, but like him I wasn't sure.

———————

When I asked the resident if she'd noticed Jessie's low sodium level, she admitted she hadn't. I gave her full marks for honesty. The resident stifled a yawn. "You're allowed to be tired," I told her. She smiled a sheepish grin, as if she'd been caught being human. She's hardly the first resident caught looking fatigued on the job.

"On average, residents typically work a minimum of sixty hours up to a maximum of eighty hours a week," said Dr. Roona Sinha on

White Coat, Black Art. At the time, Dr. Sinha was a resident in pediatric hematology and oncology (blood disorders and cancer in children) and recent president of the Canadian Association of Interns and Residents, the body that represents the more than 7,500 residents across the country. "But residents in some programs work up to one hundred hours a week."

Think that's a lot? It used to be considerably worse. When I was a first-year resident at the Hospital for Sick Children in Toronto in 1980, I was on-call one night in three. On average, I worked seventy to eighty hours a week. If I was on-call for an entire weekend, it was more like 110 hours. The nights on-call were seldom easy or stress-free. When babies get sick, you pull out all the stops to save them. Add to that the challenge of taking blood, starting intravenous drips and doing spinal taps on screaming toddlers—as their anxious mothers look on—and you can begin to see why I seldom if ever slept during those nights on-call. Then there were the weekends. For one entire weekend every month, I was on-call. That meant I went to work dark and early on Friday morning and didn't step out into the night sky until six the following Monday night.

In 1980, the pediatric cardiology service at the Hospital for Sick Children moved into the newly built wards 4A and 4B. Coincidentally, I began my first year of residency at the hospital in July 1980, and for my first rotation, I was assigned to 4B. My senior resident was George Rutherford III, who has had a long and distinguished career as a specialist in public health. Currently, he is the director of the Institute for Global Health and head of the division of Preventive Medicine and Public Health at the University of California, San Francisco (UCSF).

Back then, Rutherford was an American from UCSF who had come to Sick Kids, known then (as now) as one of the top pediatric hospitals in the world, to round out his American education with "international" experience. He was smart, suave and worldly-wise. He had one additional qualification that made him one of the coolest guys I'd ever known. Back in his undergraduate days at UCSF, he was a teammate of tennis legend Jimmy Connors on the collegiate team.

Rutherford had a dry, WASPish sense of humour that took a young, Jewish and highly neurotic junior resident like me a little getting used to. Following my first night on call, Rutherford arrived on the ward, saw my haggard appearance, not to mention the "deer in the headlights" look in my eyes, and made a beeline for me.

"So, Brian," he asked, putting a reassuring hand on my shoulder, "how many did you box last night?" Box, as in coffin. He wanted to know how many patients I'd killed! For a half-second, he kept a perfectly deadpan look on his face before breaking out into a big grin. It was easy to pull my leg back in those days.

As I struggled to survive my gruelling residency, I never thought to question why I had to put in more than a hundred hours in a week. That we ask it today—let alone put a stop to it—is an indication of how much things have changed.

There is a culture in medicine that says physicians are supposed to suffer as a rite of passage. To earn membership in the club, mentors expect residents to be able to work long hours and endure sleep deprivation, just as they had to prove to their mentors a generation ago. And so on.

As I said, when I was a resident, I was on-call one night in three. Before my time, it was one night in two. Every concession to human fatigue and frailty was greeted with sarcastic derision. A veteran surgeon once told me: "You know the problem with working on-call one night in two? You miss half the great cases."

We were supposed to work hard and to suffer in silence. To complain was to show weakness. If you were training to be a surgeon, your mentors would wonder whether you had the stamina to do the job. Even today, that's still the case.

"If you complain or try to stand up for your right to go home, attendings [the physicians on duty] wonder if you've got what it takes," said Dr. Roona Sinha on *White Coat, Black Art.* "You may be subjected to intimidation and psychological and even physical abuse." She says the physical abuse might include having sharp surgical instruments handed to you in an inappropriate way during an operation.

It took the death of an eighteen-year-old college freshman named Libby Zion to bring the issue of overwork and sleep deprivation under the spotlight. On the evening of March 4, 1984, Zion was admitted to New York Hospital with a high fever and jerking movements. Her only other medical problem was a history of depression, for which her family doctor prescribed phenelzine, an antidepressant.

Residents contacted Zion's family physician and decided to admit Zion with a diagnosis of a possible viral infection. Zion was given intravenous fluids and injections of meperidine (also known as Demerol) to help control her shaking. It was 3:00 a.m. when she was admitted to hospital.

Over the next few hours, Zion became more agitated. The residents on-call who admitted Zion ordered physical restraints as well as an injection of haloperidol, a sedative used in psychotic patients who are agitated. By 6:00 a.m., Zion was calmer, but her temperature had risen to nearly 42 degrees Celsius (107.6 degrees Fahrenheit). Soon after, she suffered cardiac arrest, and could not be resuscitated.

Zion's family sued the hospital for negligence. The father, Sidney Zion, a former lawyer and journalist, persuaded the Manhattan district attorney to convene a grand jury to consider murder charges against the residents. Ultimately, the residents were never charged.

However, the grand jury issued a report that was scathing in its criticism of work schedules of residents, in particular the tendency for residents to have to work up to thirty-six hours at a stretch.

The problem still exists. A study published in 2006 in the *Public Library of Science* (PLoS) by Laura K. Barger and colleagues at the Brigham and Women's Hospital in Boston found that residents who worked five or more extended duration or "marathon" shifts (defined as thirty hours or more in duration) were seven times more likely to report at least one medical error related to fatigue. As well, fatigue-related preventable mistakes associated with the death of the patient increased threefold.

A state commission headed by New York physician Dr. Bertrand Bell recommended that residents work no more than eighty hours a week and no more than twenty-four hours in a row. In 2003, the Accreditation Council for Graduate Medical Education made mandatory the same recommendations for all residency programs in the United States. In December 2008, the Institute of Medicine released a report entitled "Resident Duty Hours: Enhancing Sleep, Supervision, and Safety," in which it recommended no more than sixteen hours of scheduled continuous duty, unless a five-hour period of uninterrupted continuous sleep is provided between 10:00 p.m. and 8:00 a.m. The institute also adopted the maximum eighty hours of work per week recommended by Dr. Bell in the New York state commission report.

In Canada, provincial associations of interns and residents, which are in effect the unions representing residents, have negotiated reductions in the number of hours residents are permitted to work before they must be allowed to go home. For instance, as of July 1, 2009, residents in Ontario are permitted to be on-call no more than every fourth night. And they are permitted to go home from the hospital by 8:00 a.m. the morning following the on-call, or up to an hour or an hour and a half later, depending on the residency program.

The rules are a lot more humane than in my time as a resident. But even though residents may be permitted to go home, many fail to exercise that right. I found that out when I interviewed a group of residents from Ontario. As I write this, all of them are still in residency, and at risk of being washed out of their programs for speaking up. So I've protected their identities.

"It happens all the time," said one of the residents. "There's no way around it. If you walk away, you let your patient down. That's a huge factor."

"The public might be surprised to know that in some areas, particularly surgical rotations, residents going to the operating room to assist in surgery will have already been up for more than a full day—people doing or assisting with brain surgery or hip replacements," another ER resident said.

"I remember doing that in medical school, having been up all night and being asked to stay and help in surgery the next day," he added. "You leave to go home and you jeopardize the operation taking place, and so you get a bad evaluation from your attending."

The scary thing is that even today, with all the talk of making schedules more humane than in my day, sleep deprivation is still a big problem among residents.

A couple of years ago, I shadowed Heather Wilson, at the time a fifth-year surgical resident at Dalhousie University in Halifax, along with her team of junior residents. I asked her the longest stretch of time she'd worked as a resident.

"I don't know. Thirty-six or thirty-eight hours," she told me on *White Coat, Black Art.* "I've been on-call for an entire weekend, but I've never been up straight that long. I'm sure there are people out there who have been. I'm fortunate to not be one of them."

How did she function at the thirty-six- or thirty-eight-hour mark? "You know, I don't think you ever really think you're that impaired when you're in the midst of it," she said. "I think the nice thing about being in the hospital is that there are a lot of safeguards in place. I mean, when you write drug orders, there's a pharmacist checking them. They're not going to send up something that's dangerous to the patient. And similarly with the nurses, if you ask them to do something unreasonable or unsafe, or if you ask them to do it for the wrong patient or something like that, there are checks in the system that should prevent it from hitting the patient."

Of course, that is if the nurses and pharmacists who do the checking are more rested than the residents.

Once, I worked a night shift with a third-year resident in emergency medicine. It was five-thirty in the morning and both of us were tired. He had seen a patient with a dark spot in the centre of her vision. From my resident's description, it sounded like the patient either had a retinal detachment or a vitreous hemorrhage. In either case, we needed to get a better look at the patient's retina. In those situations, we use drops to dilate the pupil.

"Are these the drops I'm supposed to put in?" the resident asked as he handed over a container. I looked at the label and saw that the dropper contained pilocarpine, a medication that constricts rather than dilates the pupil.

"Don't use pilocarpine," I told him. I even took him to the cart in the eye room where I showed him the drops to use. "Here," I said, opening up the drawers as I spoke. "Put one drop of phenyl-ephrine and one drop of cyclopentolate into the eye."

First, I showed the resident how to test the patient's eye for glaucoma before putting in drops to dilate the pupil. That's a necessary precaution, since dilating a pupil of a patient with glaucoma can make the pressure in the eye rise dangerously and cause permanent damage.

The pressure in the eye was normal. Then it was time for my resident to put the drops in to dilate the pupil. He put in the cyclopentolate. But when he reached into the drawer for phenylephrine he didn't notice that he had once again grabbed a dropper that contained pilocarpine. He noticed his mistake only after he'd put the wrong drops into my patient's eye. And this was after I'd taken the time to explain which drops to put in and why. Fortunately, there were no serious consequences. At worst, the drop of pilocarpine counteracted the dilating effect of cyclopentolate and phenylephrine. Still, it made me realize that my resident was tired and sleep deprived. And error prone.

In the ER, I was able to catch that mistake because I'm always on hand when I'm on duty. However, unless the resident tells me what he's about to do, there's no way I'm going to be able to catch everything. If I second-guessed every history, every physical, every test and every treatment by a resident, I'd still be at the hospital trying to finish my first shift.

There are fixes out there to help residents have shorter, more humane work schedules. The system could hire more nurse practitioners and physician assistants to take away some of the scut work we pile on residents. Scut work refers to chores that residents have to do that take up time and don't add to the educational experience. Filling out forms and other clerical work come to mind immediately.

Some countries have cut back on the number of hours a resident is allowed to work each week. But the price is that residents get less experience, or they need several more years to complete their education. Many of the residents I've spoken with aren't interested in that idea. "I would personally dread coming to work knowing that I was still going to be training for the next ten, fifteen years," Dr. Heather Wilson says. "I think you would lose a lot of people along the way."

Whether you agree or disagree with Wilson, you've got to admire her honesty.

2:42 A.M.

The resident and I sat down to talk about how to manage Jessie and her low sodium level, then the resident went off to see another patient. I thought about Jessie. On the one hand, this kind of case is where I really earn my pay. Jessie started out as a straightforward Tylenol overdose. But a little voice in the back of my head told me to probe deeper. When I found the abnormal sodium level, I was satisfied we'd discovered the real cause of Jessie's symptoms. She'd be admitted to hospital but would soon recover.

At the same time, I felt uneasy about the way I'd discovered the low sodium level. Had the department been busier, and the resident more confident in her judgment, I might not have insisted on seeing Jessie and checking the blood tests myself.

It's happened before, and I'm quite sure it will happen again.

CHAPTER SEVEN

ZONKED IN THE NIGHT

2:42 A.M.

I had slept for an hour at the most before coming on duty, a fitful nap after getting home from a long day at the CBC. It wasn't unusual for me to be functioning on minimal rest. I've been operating this way for a long time, juggling two careers and, since meeting Tamara, trying to be a good husband and father to our children. I've always had a lot of energy and the ability to suppress the voices inside my head telling me to give in to my exhaustion. Giving up on what I'm supposed to be doing has never been an option.

I guess it's because I'm blessed—some might say cursed—with the skill and energy to pursue more than one career path at the same time. For some MDs, being an emergency physician is all they ever wanted. Not for me. For one thing, I started working in the ER to give myself time to write. Truth is, I also like having two careers because I don't feel as much pressure to be the best at either. A wise person once gave me this useful piece of advice: "If you can't be the best be different."

When I have a bad day at the CBC, I take solace in reminding myself that I also practise emergency medicine. When I have a difficult shift at Mount Sinai, I remind myself that I'm one of very few ER physicians with a career in radio.

The other thing about having two careers is that the variety of experiences keeps me from getting bored. It's no accident I stayed with emergency medicine—no two shifts are alike.

Everyone talks about the adrenaline rush of working in the ER. No doubt it's there, but I don't feel it like I used to. Maybe it's a function of getting older. I think there's something else that drives doctors and nurses to the ER that no one talks about. We tend to have short attention spans. Some of us probably have undiagnosed attention deficit hyperactivity disorder (ADHD). Our brains need constant stimulation to keep us engaged. If the ER grinds to a halt because no patients are arriving, our minds start to wander.

In practical terms, we're really good at what's called episodic care. That means seeing patients once for a medical problem. Someone comes in with a kidney stone, a sore throat or a sprained ankle. I treat the problem and send the patient on her way. What we aren't good at is what's known as continuing care—seeing a patient in the ER through an illness that lasts several days or perhaps even longer.

"What are we doing with this patient?" a nurse recently asked me. I picked up the chart and groaned. That question is usually the first clue that we have a patient who is at risk of falling through the cracks. An eighty-nine-year-old woman named Chaya had been in our ER for seventy-two hours waiting for a bed at a rehabilitation facility. (We often hold patients like Chaya for two, three, even four days, often in a corridor of the ER, while a social worker arranges for the next available bed in a long-term care facility. We call that "placement.") She had fallen at home and fractured her acetabulum, the socket that forms part of the hip joint. As I quickly scanned the chart, I noticed with amazement that she hadn't had any blood tests. Why amazement? Because it seems to me we do blood tests on just about everybody, except for people with minor complaints like sprained ankles and cuts.

To us, the episode that brought the person to the ER and that we relish diagnosing—in this case, the fractured acetabulum—is over. The ER physician who makes the diagnosis writes what we call holding orders, everything from how often the nurse is supposed to take the patient's vital signs to what medications to give. Hate to say it, but once that happens, the patient ceases to be interesting to most ER physicians I know. With new patients arriving by the hour, it's easy to pass an entire shift without visiting a patient being held for placement even once. Because we work shifts, the patient gets handed from one ER physician to the next—at Sinai, that's five different physicians on a weekday. None of us acts as the attending doctor (meaning the one primarily responsible). It's as if the patient becomes part of the furniture.

I noticed that Chaya was taking a large number of medications, including a diuretic (what is referred to commonly as a water pill) for heart failure. "Let's get some blood work," I told the nurse. Good thing I did. Her serum sodium was abnormally low at 118 milliequivalents per litre. When I got the lab result, I smiled for a couple of reasons. The first was that the low sodium may have helped explain why Chaya had fallen and broken her acetabulum. A low sodium causes dehydration, and dehydration causes dizziness, which can lead to falls. The second was that the low sodium gave me a plausible reason to refer Chaya for admission to the internal medicine team. That got Chaya out of the corridor and into a hospital bed.

Still, I was troubled by the fact that several ER colleagues and I had essentially ignored her. As the physician on duty, I was responsible for her welfare. Patients like Chaya are just one more reason why I worry when I go home following a shift.

_____

The downside of having two busy careers is that I try to pack too much into my days. Everyone who works nights has a different routine. Ideally, you get to sleep in late the morning prior to your first night. Not a chance with me, since I work days at the CBC. Even if I didn't, I have a lifelong tendency to wake up early in the morning. Besides, on weekdays, when Tamara sets the alarm for 6:20 a.m., I usually get up with the alarm. I'm seldom able to get back to sleep.

Some of my colleagues are able to nap for two or three hours during the afternoon or evening prior to the first night. I've always been able to nap, but seldom longer than forty-five minutes to an hour. In general, how rested I am depends largely on how well I've been sleeping in the days prior to the night shift. I'm a worrywart by nature. Crisis at the CBC, a problem with one of my kids, a roof that needs fixing, you name it. There's always something that keeps my mind racing first thing in the morning and often keeps me from sleeping well.

In the past, I got anxious about working at night when I knew I hadn't been sleeping well and felt tired. It was bad enough that I didn't feel rested. Compounding that was the fear that fatigue and sleep deprivation would take away my alertness and increase the likelihood of making mistakes on the job.

This is no idle concern. According to the U.S. National Highway Traffic Safety Administration, it is conservatively estimated that 100,000 of the motor vehicle collisions a year that are reported to the police are directly attributable to driver fatigue. There are fears the real number is far larger. Using data from recent epidemio-logical studies, the U.S. Institute of Medicine estimates that as many as one million motor vehicle collisions, 500,000 injures and 8,000 fatalities a year on U.S. roads may be due to drowsiness caused by sleep deprivation.

Numerous manmade disasters, including the nuclear accident at Three Mile Island, the nuclear meltdown at Chernobyl, the explo-sion of the space shuttle *Challenger* and the *Exxon Valdez* oil spill were caused at least in part by sleep deprivation.

Frankly, you'd have to be a fool to believe that health profes-sionals are immune to the effects of sleep deprivation. But you rarely hear my colleagues talking about how tired they feel doing nights, and how it affects their performance on the job.

Dr. Steven Park, a New York surgeon and author of *Sleep, Inter-rupted: A Physician Reveals the #1 Reason Why So Many of Us Are Sick and Tired,* recalls vividly the month he did an ER rotation dur-ing his internship year. "I was on rotating 8-hour shifts, which lasted one week at a time," he writes. "After completing one 10 pm to 6 am shift, as I was driving home, I nodded off and had to swerve suddenly to avoid hitting an oncoming car at 50 miles per hour. I'd been used to regular shifts where I went 36 to 40 hours being on-call for my regular surgical rotations, but this was the first time I had ever experienced a rotating shift. I almost died that morning."

Park cites studies that illustrate how normal shift work, never mind the yo-yo schedule I am often on, results in increased acci-dents, increased health problems such as cancer, heart disease and depression, and social stresses from reduced interactions with family and friends.

I see and experience the effects of sleep deprivation all the time. Sometimes when I'm speaking to a nurse, I find myself substitut-ing one word for another. Not long ago, I saw a patient in alcohol withdrawal. I asked the nurse to give the patient a dose of diazepam, a drug we administer to get rid of the shakes. At least, that's what I thought I was saying. Turns out my sleep-deprived brain asked instead for diltiazem, a drug used to slow the heart rate of patients with an irregular heart rhythm called atrial fibrillation.

Fortunately, the strange look on the nurse's face made me quickly aware of my mistake. My patient got diazepam as intended. If the nurse had followed my original order for diltiazem the drug would have lowered my patient's blood pressure, perhaps dangerously so.

Sometimes, the effects of sleep deprivation can be amusing in a weird sort of way. One night, about twenty years ago, I was working with a resident in family medicine. Her personality was anal-retentive and she possessed an encyclopedic knowledge of medicine. She tended to pad her histories with far more medical information than needed to make a quick diagnosis.

Around 5:00 a.m., she came to my office to tell me about a patient with a sore throat. The patient was middle-aged, and free of serious medical problems. Instead of zeroing in on the sore throat and whether or not to prescribe antibiotics, the resident presented the patient's normal medical history in exhaustive detail. From birth. Around four or five minutes into the history, my eyes started to get heavy. I found myself trying to stay awake during her long and laborious litany of normal findings. Right hand underneath the desktop and out of sight of the resident, I grasped my thigh and pinched it harder and harder in an effort to stay awake, but to no avail. The last thought I had was, what else can I do next to keep myself awake? And then . . .

Darkness.

The next thing I knew the resident was shaking my shoulders to rouse me. I had fallen asleep while listening to her describe a patient. Embarrassed? You bet. And mostly because I had been busted demonstrating a human frailty. In medicine, there's an unwritten rule that you're not supposed to be bothered by the things that affect mere mortals. If you're sick, you're supposed to suck it up and come to work, although you should wear a surgical mask if you've got a cold. If you're sued for negligence, don't tell a judge or jury you missed that blood clot in the lungs because you were busy running three cardiac arrests simultaneously. And if you make a mistake, don't ever admit that sleep deprivation played a role.

This attitude is emblematic of the time-honoured culture of medicine, and the ER is no exception. If anything, the issue of sleep deprivation is much bigger in the ER than it is in many other areas of hospital medicine. Doctors in specialties like general surgery and internal medicine work regular weekday hours, say 7:00 a.m. or 8:00 a.m. to 5:00 p.m. or 6:00 p.m., Monday to Friday. As for nights and weekends, one attending surgeon or internist is on-call and available to take care of patients on the wards as well as newly referred patients in the ER. On a busy night, the attending physician may be up for hours, but between calls, he or she can go to sleep, often at home. Since they usually work only one night on-call at a time, most attending physicians feel quite capable of working the next day, especially if they work at a teaching hospital and have residents at the ready to take care of most problems.

Emergency physicians are almost unique in the world of medicine. When we're scheduled to work at night, we do exactly that. Like nurses and other shift workers, we're expected to function during the entire night as if it's daytime; whether we're able to or not is an altogether different question. Anaesthetists, critical care specialists and even obstetricians at some hospitals have begun working twelve-hour shifts.

I did my first shift at Mount Sinai Hospital's ER on February 28, 1984. Although I had some sense of life in an ER from my previous experiences, jumping into it full-time proved incredibly taxing. I had no idea I would find the long hours and relentless pressure to treat the endless flow of patients so difficult. What I found especially gruelling was the erratic shift schedule. I knew from my medical training and days as an intern and resident that our circadian rhythms—our biological clock, so to speak—were disturbed by shift work. I just had no idea how intense the effects could be when the shift work fluctuated as much as it did for an ER doctor.

Typically, I would work four days in a row from Tuesday to Friday from 7:00 a.m. to 3:00 p.m., although it was rarely possible to leave that early. Most shifts would last ten to eleven hours because you couldn't just walk out the door—at least I couldn't—when there were patients I had started to treat during my shift who had not yet reached a certain point of completion. If I'd ordered blood work for someone who could be suffering from several potential problems, for example, I found it impossible to just hand the patient over to the physician replacing me. I needed to see the results and talk further with the patient and possibly family members and friends before my conscience let me head out the door. Also, I found that as the time for the new doc to arrive got closer, my histories and physicals got quicker and less comprehensive. I was embarrassed to hand these patients over to the next colleague because I was afraid he or she would see immediately what a shoddy workup I'd done.

Following the Tuesday to Friday rotation I'd have the weekend off and return Monday at 3:00 p.m. for a shift that officially ended at 11:00 that night. I'd do the same on Tuesday and Wednesday. Thursday would be off. I'd then come in Friday, Saturday and Sunday for the overnight shift, which ran, in theory, from 7:30 p.m. to 7:00 a.m. The next five days would be off, followed by a 7:00 a.m. to 7:30 p.m. shift on the Saturday, Sunday and Monday. The next two days would be off, then I'd be back in for an afternoon shift on

Thursday and Friday. I'd be off Saturday and Sunday but back on nights for Monday through Thursday. And so on. Although I'd get a sixteen-day break every seven weeks, the constant change in the hours of work made this challenging new job even more difficult to manage.

The jitterbug nature of my work schedule—not to mention added duties such as teaching and committee work—reinforced my insomnia. I had battled insomnia during certain periods of my childhood, so I was already prone to this affliction. Not surprisingly, it resurfaced not long into my inaugural stint at Mount Sinai. I found myself operating on about four hours' sleep a night, which after a few weeks put me into a cloudy state.

I will never forget the time I misdiagnosed two patients who turned out to have appendicitis. One I thought had a kidney stone, the other an intestinal infection. At the end of my shift, I handed over both patients to a colleague who had come on for the day shift. For the patient with the suspected kidney infection, I had ordered an intravenous pyelogram (IVP), in which dye is injected into the body and followed through the kidneys to identify a blockage caused by a stone. When the IVP was normal, which meant there was no stone, the physician to whom I'd entrusted my patient's care re-examined him rather than sending him home. He found the appendicitis. In the second case, I'd asked my colleague to reassess the patient after the blood tests I'd ordered for what I thought was the infection came back. Like the first patient, the second one turned out to have appendicitis too.

Don't for a moment think these misdiagnoses happen only to incompetent doctors. At one time or another, they happen to all of us. A few years ago, I was working a day shift when a very experienced colleague asked me to look after a patient he'd seen in the middle of a very busy night shift. The patient, a man in his eighties, had come in with abdominal pain. This was his second visit to the ER in a week. On the first, he had a CT scan of his abdomen, which was normal, and he was discharged. A week later, he returned with pain that had become worse. My colleague, who had seen the man during the night, had given him some morphine to relieve his pain and said he thought he would be able to go home a few hours later. Something in the patient's symptoms made me think this was wrong: his abdomen was tender, and he was vomiting bile.

As I started asking more and more questions about the patient, my colleague thought better of his plan to discharge him. Instead, he ordered a second CT scan of the abdomen. This one showed that the patient had several feet of dead small bowel in his small intestine, caused by a condition called ischemic colitis. He needed emergency surgery. If I'd followed my colleague's original advice and discharged him, our patient would almost certainly have died within several hours.

Diagnostic errors happen all the time. My failure to diagnose the two appendicitis cases caught the attention of the chief of the ER, Howard Ovens, who called me to task. "I want to know how you were doing that night because some of the nurses said you looked tired," he said. "I consider fatigue as a form of impairment." His tone was reprimanding, with a slight edge of anxiety, as if he was trying to press a point. Impairment is a loaded term. It suggests drunkenness or sloppiness. It says you can't manage your sleep. It says you can't manage yourself. Needless to say, I was mortified and ashamed. I am easily shaken by any criticism, and this one pierced deeply into my psyche. Although every doctor has experiences such as mine, it was hard for me, especially when I was relatively new to the hospital, to allow myself that weakness.

No matter what caused me to misdiagnose the patients, I knew that fatigue was an issue I had to address. Desperate for a solution,

I signed up for a sleep electroencephalogram (EEG) at the sleep laboratory at Toronto Western Hospital, where the sleep specialist suggested I try taking amitriptyline, an antidepressant that is used to treat migraines and, in small doses such as twenty-five milligrams, works as a sleeping pill. That brought some immediate help falling asleep, although I would still wake up at five in the morning and have trouble getting back to sleep, usually because I had too much on my mind. Ten years ago, my physician switched me from amitriptyline to a small dose of mirtazapine, which works better.

The one sleep aid I absolutely avoid is sleeping pills. Funny, because in the ER we dole out lorazepam like candy to psych patients. Lorazepam is a benzodiazepine, the same class of drugs that includes diazepam, or Valium (once known as "mother's little helper" because of the tendency of physicians to prescribe it to housewives back in the 1960s and 1970s). Lorazepam is used in the short-term management of anxiety. Benzodiazepines have long been prescribed by doctors as sleeping pills. But they can lead to addiction, as well as cognitive and memory impairment.

Memory problems were brought a little too close to home with a study published in the *Journal of Emergency Medicine* in 1989. At the time, triazolam, sold under the brand name Halcion, was prescribed as a sleeping pill. ER physicians took triazolam to help them get to sleep in the hours before a shift. However, J. Stephen Huff and Harry G. Plunkett published a case report of two emergency physicians who took triazolam at bedtime and experienced profound amnesia in the ER the next day. One of the physicians reported that he went through an entire shift seeing patients and prescribing treatments and later had almost no recall of any of the patients he had seen.

To stay awake at night, I have often relied on caffeine. I sometimes bring to work a large single-cream double-sugar from Tim Hortons, along with a box of forty Timbits. The people I work with at night are always grateful for food, garbage calories aside. But I've long found that while one cup of coffee increases my alertness, any more tends to make me antsy without improving my wakefulness or my ability to think. I became resigned to feeling somewhat impaired at night.

Then I discovered modafinil.

Modafinil is sold under the brand names Alertec and Provigil. The drug was first approved in 1998 by the U.S. Food and Drug Administration and in 1999 by Health Canada for the treatment of narcolepsy, a neurological sleep disorder characterized by uncontrollable attacks of daytime sleepiness. Modafinil is a mild stimulant that works by increasing the release of the chemicals norepinephrine and dopamine in the brain areas associated with euphoria or pleasure. The drug also raises the level of histamine inside a part of the brain called the hypothalamus. It's this effect that has led some researchers to postulate that modafinil is less a stimulant than a drug that promotes wakefulness.

With fewer than 24,000 Canadians suffering from narcolepsy, modafinil was hardly destined to become a blockbuster like the latest cholesterol-lowering drugs. But something happened to make the drug go viral.

Although modafinil was approved originally as a treatment for narcolepsy, there's nothing to stop doctors from prescribing it or any other drug for any indication for which there is at least some clinical evidence of efficacy. That is known as "off-label" prescribing. A growing number of regulators and other authorities condemn off-label prescribing as little more than a vehicle by which pharmaceutical companies can drive up sales. There are efforts underway to eliminate off-label prescribing.

That said, some of the early narcoleptics who used modafinil found they made smoother transitions to various shifts. It wasn't long before doctors started prescribing the drug to a small number of patients who complained bitterly of excessive sleepiness during night shifts. Then Charles Czeisler, a leading sleep researcher from Harvard Medical School, and his colleagues put modafinil to the test. They recruited 209 patients with shift-work sleep disorder and randomly assigned test subjects to receive either 200 milligrams of modafinil or a placebo at the start of each shift. Subjects kept a diary of how they performed at work and were sent for numerous wakefulness tests. Compared with subjects given the placebo, those treated with modafinil were more wakeful and experienced a small but significant improvement in performance of their duties. The study was published in the *New England Journal of Medicine* in 2005.

With that, off-label prescribing of the drug increased significantly. In 2006, Health Canada extended the approval of modafinil to include patients with excessive sleepiness in shift work. Then, Michael Gill and colleagues pitted modafinil against a placebo in a study of sleep-deprived emergency physicians. Modafinil improved cognitive performance, augmented working memory and perceived alertness, and reduced mental errors.

Tellingly, the U.S. military found modafinil beneficial in Iraq. "Soldiers can stay awake and function alertly for 40 hours, get eight hours of sleep, and then stay awake for 40 more, all without the impaired judgment of old-fashioned uppers," the *Ottawa Citizen* reported in October 2003.

As soon as I started taking modafinil, I found it a godsend. It increases my alertness by about 10 to 20 percent. And it does so without giving me the antsiness I used to get from coffee. Still, if all it did was keep me alert, I probably wouldn't bother taking it. Like many others, though, I've noticed something else. I'm more focused. I can remember more things and I can synthesize more medical facts.

And I'm not alone. Modafinil has joined the ranks of what are known as cognitive enhancers. Another drug used as a cognitive enhancer is methylphenidate, also known as Ritalin, which is prescribed to patients with ADHD. In the U.S., some colleges report rates of methylphenidate use as high as 25 percent.

As off-label use of modafinil took off, reports of side effects increased. They include headaches (I get a mild headache on occasion), severe skin reactions and worsening of psychiatric symptoms. It should be avoided in patients with certain heart conditions and is not approved for children. Because it enhances dopamine release, there are concerns it might be habit forming.

So, is modafinil like steroids to a major league baseball player or like those high-tech swimsuits that in 2009 enabled swimmers to demolish world records? Maybe, but let me ask you this: do you want me clean, or do you want me to know the difference between diazepam and diltiazem? Thought so.

2:44 A.M.

I took a modafinil and headed to my next patient, Alexei, an elderly man who had fainted in a hotel bar a few hours earlier. He was eighty-two and in reasonable condition, with type 2 diabetes his only apparent medical concern. The nurses noted he had been complaining non-stop since being brought in by paramedics that he was fine and just wanted to go home. His blood work showed his blood sugar levels to be slightly elevated but not to any alarming degree. He had a little alcohol in his system but again nothing to warrant concern. Sadly, to me at least, he lived alone and had no immediate family.

To be truthful, this was the last kind of case I wanted to deal with at a quarter to three in the morning as I struggled with fatigue.

Unless I discovered something unforeseen, it was more than likely a routine matter that ate up time and energy and offered little in return to get my creative juices flowing, which was what my system needed to re-energize me.

Alexei was about six feet tall and a good thirty or more pounds overweight, most of it parked around his belly. He had a slight Russian accent and a sneering disposition. As soon as I entered his room and introduced myself, he announced he was fine and demanded to be sent home. I told him that before I could release him I needed to make sure he was all right.

"What happened to you tonight?" I asked.

"I fainted. No big anything. Shit happens, eh?"

"Why were you at the hotel?"

"None of your goddamn business," he said, a slight and cocky grin on his face. I've noticed that more patients swear at doctors these days than when I first started in medicine.

"Why are you grinning?" I asked. Some doctors might not have noticed the way he punctuated his response. If they did, they might not have considered it meaningful or something they had a right to comment on. I have studied human behaviour throughout my life and am hypersensitive to the way people speak. I'm especially sensitive to their non-verbal communication; I know it usually reveals more than what they actually say. I also trust my instincts, and in this case they were telling me to probe a bit more deeply into his answer.

"Maybe I was meeting someone."

"At the bar?"

"Yeah. Why not? I'm old, not dead. Not yet anyway."

It dawned on me that if he were twenty or more years younger I would likely assume, from his vagueness, that his rendezvous was with a woman. "A lady?" I asked.

"Very good," he said proudly. And then the story came out. The woman in question was a working girl he'd contacted via the Internet. His plan was to meet her at the bar and then book a room for a few hours. Unfortunately for Alexei, when the young woman saw him at the hotel she refused to go through with the transaction.

"She said I was too old. She was worried I'd die on her if we . . . you know. Said it happened to one of her friends and the police came and lots of trouble. I finished my drink and got up and next I know I'm on the ground passed out. From lack of excitement probably." He let out a deep laugh that made his belly wobble. "Now you know everything and I can go home, right?"

I was starting to like Alexei. But I wasn't ready to check him out. I asked him a series of questions to assess his competence.

"Do you know where you are?" He knew he was in hospital but couldn't tell me which one.

He didn't know the day but he nailed the month. "You always know what day it is?" he asked. I didn't answer but admitted to myself that sometimes I didn't.

"When was the last time you saw a doctor?"

"Years ago," he said. "I don't remember. Not long enough as far as I'm concerned."

"Have you fainted before, recently?"

"No," he said. But he could have been lying.

By the end of my questions I felt he was perhaps in the early stages of some kind of dementia, but I had no medical reason to keep him at the ER. I was concerned that he lived alone, in an apartment. He said he had a kind neighbour who looked in on him. I didn't think it was right that someone his age apparently had no family members to care for him. I didn't know why he was alone, and it wasn't my business, although I sensed he was the kind of person who could easily alienate others. I offered to have a social worker look in on him, but he told me not to bother. As soon as I said he could go, he began to get dressed at a speed most impressive for someone his age.

"You're a nice man," he said, and offered me his hand. I shook it warmly.

Alexei passed by the main nurse's station as he headed for the exit. Somewhat against my better judgment I asked him whether he had any children who might look in on him.

"I told you. No next of kin," he said brusquely. Then he added: "Not any I want to see or want to see me." As he left to get into a waiting cab I felt a wave of sadness overcome me. I couldn't imagine anything much worse than being old and disconnected from my children. That thought was front of mind when I saw my next patient, a single mother whose two-year-old son had what she thought was a bad cold.

After examining the boy's chest and lungs I told her I was quite certain he had pneumonia. A look of panic came into her eyes. She was a big woman with an open-hearted face. "I always make him wear the right amount of clothes. I never—"

I cut her off. The boy looked well taken care of and happy and comfortable with his mother. She was in the ER alone in the middle of the night. Another person who should have had someone with her.

"It's okay," I said. "You've done nothing wrong." My instincts told me there was a lot behind that panicked reaction. They also told me she was probably doing her best with a lot on her plate. "You're a good mother. You brought your child in here as soon as you felt something was wrong. Lots of kids get pneumonia. It's not a sign of neglect. We'll get some antibiotics in him and he'll be his normal self before you know it. He'll also likely sleep well when you get him home."

As I got up to write out the prescription I touched her gently on the shoulder, a reassuring pat. "You get some sleep," I said. She smiled and nodded. I doubt she knew how well I understood the need for sleep. All of us who work the night shift know that only too well. What I needed now was a really engaging case.

CHAPTER EIGHT

I NEVER FORGET THE NAMES
OF THOSE WHO DIE

3:02 A.M.

When I was a child, broken telephone was one of my favourite class-room games. Also known as Chinese whispers, whispers down the line, and Arab phone, broken telephone is a party game in which one person invents a story and then whispers it to the person beside him. That person recounts it to the next player, and she does the same to the next and so on, until everyone has had the story spoken into their ear. At the end the original and the final version are com-pared. They are rarely, if ever, the same.

But that's a game. In real life, broken telephone is a challenge ER doctors like me have to deal with. When the story changes, someone's life can be on the line.

In the ER, a patient will often describe her circumstances to four or five people: the paramedics, a triage nurse, a nurse working on the floor, a resident, a specialist and, of course, an ER doctor. It's not unusual for the patient to keep changing the story for several reasons, one being the desire to please the person asking the questions. "You seem to be touching your abdomen a lot," the triage nurse will notice. "Does it hurt there?" The patient nods. Ah, a case of abdominal pain. Then the resident shows up in the patient's room an hour later. "Do you have chest pains?" the resident asks. The patient again nods. Now we have two differing symptoms. I see the patient forty-five minutes after that. "Where does it hurt?" I'll ask. "I'm not sure," the patient might answer, "but my lower back is killing me."

The more vague and subjective the symptom, the more open it is to suggestion. The vaguest symptom by far in clinical medicine is dizziness. (I know more than my fair share about the subject. I've written a chapter on dizziness that appeared in the three most recent editions of a standard textbook of emergency medicine found in ERs across North America and around the world.)

Just for fun, go to an ER and tell the triage nurse or the emergency doctor you have dizziness and watch their faces. If they don't flinch or sigh, I'll buy you a coffee. Dizziness is one symptom that drives the people who work in the ER crazy. Or dizzy. Or both. That's because dizziness, like pain, is a subjective experience that you feel inside your head. Unless I can climb inside your head and feel it too, I'm depending on your giving me an accurate description of what you're feeling.

About twenty years ago, I woke up in a hotel room in New York City, stretched my arms, looked up at the ceiling, and turned my head a bit to look at a cockroach on the wall. Suddenly, I felt like I was on a merry-go-round. The walls started spinning. I broke out in cold sweat, got nauseated and threw up twice. I needed to take dimenhydrinate, an over-the-counter remedy for motion sickness, just to be able to take an elevator to the coffee shop for some breakfast.

What I had was an attack of vertigo, caused by particles of calcium that were floating in my middle ear. When some patients complain of dizziness, they mean vertigo.

Trouble is, that's not every patient's definition of dizziness. For some, it means fainting or nearly fainting. For others, it means a loss of balance so severe they have trouble walking a straight line or standing without listing to one side or even falling. To patients with panic attacks or agoraphobia, dizziness is the feeling they get when overcome with symptoms of anxiety.

It's our job to figure out which is which. And the stakes can be high. If you've got vertigo, you probably need to see an ear, nose and throat surgeon. If you've fainted, maybe you have a heart rhythm disturbance and you need to see a cardiologist. Or maybe you're having a stroke and you need a CT scan and a referral to a neurologist. A referral to the wrong specialist can result in disaster.

If you think sorting this out is easy, let me tell you that dizziness is the Grand Master's version of broken telephone. I've seen four health professionals take a history of "dizziness" and come out with four different diagnoses.

It doesn't help that the desire to please contributes greatly to the potential for multiple diagnoses. So too does the human factor, the one inherent in broken telephone. As each person takes notes, the details are "whispered" along to the next person. A careless (sometimes exhausted) note taker can detail one set of symptoms; a careful note taker will have another version, and so on. I have found that a medical chart is helpful. But vulnerable as my own interpretation and listening skills are to error, nothing is a good substitute for the conversation I have with a patient or a family member who knows the patient's medical history.

I mention this because I want you to know how important it is to tell doctors and nurses the truth, as accurately as possible. If, for whatever reason, you need to change or amend your story, that's fine; it's normal. Just make sure you inform the medical professional that's what you're doing. Clear and accurate information is vital in the ER.

The information on my next patient, whom I'll call Max, was contradictory, for whatever reason, so I needed to assemble a history somewhat from scratch. Fortunately his wife, Doris, was with him and she was calm and clear.

Doris had called EMS when her husband, Max, who was in his fifties, complained he was feeling weak, drowsy and confused. I assessed him at 14 out of a possible 15 (almost full alertness) on the Glasgow Coma Scale. His chart said he had "cirrhotic liver." It turned out to be far more serious.

Doris told me he had hepatitis C, which can be acquired in various ways, although the most common is through sharing needles during illicit drug use or from having sex with a partner who has a sexually transmitted disease. Doris wasn't volunteering the source of Max's virus, and I had no need or right to ask at this point.

Max's blood work came back, and it showed he had a blood sugar count of 9.1 (normal range would be about half that). His blood pressure was 94 over 58, which is considerably low.

"Any chance Max has diabetes?" I asked.

"Oh, yes," Doris said. Either she hadn't volunteered this information or it was never entered on his chart. Nor was the fact that Max had developed sclerosis of the liver, also known as cirrhosis, as a result of the hep C. Sclerosis results from scar tissue being formed on the liver. As the scarring spreads, this vital organ starts to fail. When it does, the liver loses its ability to produce protein, fight infections, digest food and store energy. Sometimes, your kidneys fail at the same time, which makes the problem all the more life threatening. It's a serious disease that without a liver transplant is ultimately fatal.

We can pull patients back from the brink, but only if we recognize it early and treat it aggressively.

Liver failure is associated with a condition called hepatic encephalopathy, which means a brain disorder brought on by a disease of the liver. A key symptom of this condition is drowsiness during the day and wide-awake alertness at night. Typically, a person with this condition reverses the normal sleeping patterns. We call it sun-setting. "That's Max for sure," Doris confirmed.

"Raise your arms," I asked Max. When he did, I extended both his wrists and held them in that position until each wrist jerked, although not at the same time. The jerking movement is called asterixis, another sign of hepatic encephalopathy. I gamely smelled his breath to see if I detected foetor hepaticus, also known somewhat ominously as the "breath of the dead." It's a smell that's both sweet and somewhat similar to feces, a distinct aroma to say the least. One whiff and I recognized it in Max.

His collective symptoms were leading me to another diagnosis, and Doris saw something in my face, a look of concern that I betrayed.

"How bad is he?" she asked.

That's a tough question for me or any medical professional to answer. My gut told me Max was in very bad shape. But what good would it do her at that moment if I offered my opinion?

"Let me examine him a bit more first," I replied, buying some time.

Max's belly appeared pear-shaped, a telltale sign that his abdominal cavity was filled with prodigious quantities of water, something doctors refer to as ascites. I placed my middle finger on Max's abdomen and tapped on it. The sound was dull, a further indication that his belly was tense with fluid.

"Have you noticed Max's girth getting bigger?" I asked Doris.

"All of a sudden," she said. I caught a look on her face that told me she was mad at herself for not calling attention to it sooner.

I then tried to touch his liver in the right upper part of the abdomen. I could feel the liver's edge about six inches below the lowest part of the rib cage. It felt hard, and when I pressed it, Max cried out in pain. Completing my medical spadework, I gently pressed on all four quadrants of the abdomen. Max hurt when I pressed each of them; he moaned slightly from the discomfort.

I was pretty sure Max's liver was failing. Unlike with the kidneys, we don't have good blood tests to tell us if the liver is in trouble. We have to rely on indirect evidence. For instance, the liver manufactures the proteins necessary for blood to clot. If blood tests like the prothrombin time (PT) and the international normalized ratio (INR) were elevated, I could deduce that Max's liver was failing because it wasn't making enough protein factors for the blood to clot properly.

I was more concerned about the increase in Max's girth. A sudden increase in ascites in a patient like Max is often a sign that the fluid has become infected, a condition known as spontaneous bacterial peritonitis. To make the diagnosis, you have to do what's called an abdominal paracentesis, which doctors refer to colloquially as a belly tap. It's a procedure in which you put a needle in the belly cavity to take out enough fluid to test for infection. If Max had spontaneous bacterial peritonitis, we'd have to put him on intravenous antibiotics right away or he could die. If Max were more stable, I could refer him to the internal medicine service and wait for them to do the tap.

I asked the nurse looking after Max how quickly the resident in internal medicine was seeing consults. She rolled her eyes. That was as good a sign as any that the medical resident was falling further and further behind in attending to people referred by the ER. I ordered a dose of ceftriaxone, an antibiotic often given to patients with spontaneous bacterial peritonitis.

On this night, this situation was a problem not just for my patients, but for me. Here's the thing. I can consult medicine at, say, 3:00 a.m., around the time I first saw Max. But until medicine actually sees him, Max is my responsibility. And at this point, it was looking more and more like the medical resident wouldn't get round to seeing Max before a new medical team was on-call, in which case he would have to wait for the next internal medicine team at 8:00 a.m.

Max was too sick to wait. I decided to tap the belly for fluid myself, right away.

To make matters worse, I felt certain Max had hepatic encephalopathy. The classic signs were the sun-setting, wrist flapping, breath smell and ascites. To deal with the latter I froze his abdomen and slipped a needle into the lower part on the left side. I inserted a catheter into his belly and drew out about three litres of water, which was a cloudy, amber colour, likely due to an infection.

The procedure seemed to calm Max down a little and he started to drift off.

"Keep a close watch on him," I told the area nurse when we were out of earshot. "He's in rough shape. Let me know the minute anything happens."

3:18 A.M.

I left Max and went to set a broken wrist. Penny was a forty-three-year-old public relations specialist who looked far younger than her age. She had checked in a couple of hours earlier following a skateboarding accident.

"I fell off and braced my fall with my hands," she told me. "I knew I had hurt my wrist, but I thought it would be okay. After a while I got a feeling it was worse than I had realized."

Penny had been drinking with friends, she said, and decided to try skateboarding for the first time. Not surprisingly, she hadn't worn any protective equipment. Few people do, especially teenagers, who see it as uncool.

"Broken wrists are among the most common accidents for people who rollerblade, skateboard or snowboard," I said. I didn't add that she was lucky she hadn't hurt her head. She knew she had messed up—she had broken her right wrist and she was right-handed—and would have difficulty typing for at least two or three weeks or until she got the hang of hunting and pecking for computer keys without being able to bend her wrist.

Penny's wrist was swollen and bruised on the knuckle side. From the side, it looked like a dinner fork, which was a sure sign of a Colles' fracture, a term used to describe a break at the end of the radius bone, the long bone of the forearm that's on the side of the thumb. There may be an associated break at the tip of the long bone of the forearm that leads to the baby finger. This kind of break was named after Abraham Colles, an Irish surgeon who first described the injury in 1814, long before X-rays found their way into medicine.

I felt the radius at the point of maximum bruising and swelling, and Penny quickly withdrew her arm, a telltale sign of bony tenderness that almost always accompanies a break. I checked Penny's fingers to make certain they were nice and pink. I also made sure she could feel me touching her fingers and could move them. I did these tests to ensure the break hadn't damaged the arteries and the nerves in her hand.

An X-ray confirmed my suspicions. Penny had a Colles' fracture. Unfortunately, the fragment of broken radius nearest the wrist was pushed upwards and angled far out of alignment. I told Penny I'd inject some local anaesthetic to freeze the broken bones in order to perform what's called a reduction, a procedure to put the bones back into proper position. I also offered her some painkillers.

"No, thanks," she said. "I was an idiot and I deserve the pain."

I laughed and applauded her spirit, but offered again.

"I'm not used to taking medication," she said.

We get a lot of that in the ER. Many patients nowadays have a widespread suspicion of prescription medications. I told her she would make the final decision. As I headed back to my office to write up my notes, I warned myself silently to prepare for the likelihood that, without pain meds, the procedure might not go so well. That thought vanished from my mind when the nurse treating Max tracked me down.

"You better come right away," she said.

3:38 A.M.

Max had developed an upper gastrointestinal bleed. Cirrhosis predisposes patients to a condition called portal hypertension, in which the blood that normally travels through the veins of the liver instead travels through veins in the belly. As a result, patients develop huge veins called varices on the inside of the esophagus. They can start bleeding like stink, all of a sudden.

By the time I got to his room Max was vomiting pints of bright red blood that looked as if it could have been coming from the veins in his arms. He was also defecating maroon-coloured blood. Blood was coming out of both ends, and it was everywhere. A terrible mess. More to the point, Max was hemorrhaging to death. His blood pressure was dropping precipitously, and he was going into shock.

If Max was going to live, we needed to stop the bleeding. I decided quickly that he was too sick to be admitted to a general internal medicine ward. I paged the resident on-call to the intensive care unit instead. Fortunately, the resident called back within minutes.

"Did you call the GI resident?" she asked.

"Way ahead of you," I replied. "I've got GI and surgery on their way."

Some patients arrive with confusing symptoms that we have to sort out. In Max's case, there was nothing confusing about his presentation. He didn't need a diagnosis; he needed an orchestrated response to save his life. He had to be admitted to a critical care bed because, even if he survived, his life would hang in the balance for the next few days. Next, a resident plus an attending surgeon in GI (gastroenterology) needed to pass an endoscope into Max's esophagus to find the bleeding varices and inject them with sodium tetradecyl, a drug that hardens them and stops the bleeding. This procedure, called endoscopic sclerotherapy, is successful in stopping the bleeding in up to 90 percent of patients. If that fails, the next best thing is to use an endoscope to stop the bleeding by tying a rubber band around the varices. Either procedure would take time to organize.

Part of the orchestrated response was to ask the surgeons to see Max as well. Surgery is used less and less to treat patients with gastrointestinal bleeding. We now call surgeons only if the bleeding is life-threatening. If we end up needing their services, it means a patient is down to his last shot to stop the bleeding and save his life.

While all of this was going on, I had to do my bit to quickly replace the blood Max had lost—two litres and counting, by my crude estimation. We needed to pour two litres of normal saline, a salt solution necessary to fill up his arteries and veins, as quickly as possible to prevent him from going into irreversible shock. Saline was just a stop-gap. With all the blood I'd seen on the floor and on Max's bedsheets, he needed an immediate transfusion. You can't just ask for a couple of pints from the blood bank; you have to order what's called a "type and cross match." You send a vial of blood to the blood bank, where it's tested against the pints or units of blood that are being readied for transfusion to make sure they are compatible. A type and cross match takes up to an hour to perform. I wasn't sure Max had that long to live.

Besides the blood transfusion, I needed to pour two potentially life-saving drugs into Max's veins: Pantoloc (pantoprazole), a drug that reduces gastrointestinal bleeding by blocking histamine receptors that trigger acid secretion in the stomach and duodenum (part of the small intestine), and octreotide, a drug that stops bleeding by constricting the varices.

"Let's give him Pantoloc 80 milligrams bolus [a single, large quantity] and set up an 8 milligrams per hour drip," I said. "As soon as that's going, let's start a bolus of 50 micrograms of octreotide, followed by a 25 milligrams per hour drip."

There was just one problem. The transfusion, the saline and all three medications had to be given by intravenous drip. Max needed a second IV, and the nurses couldn't find a vein in which to insert one. The typical places nurses try are on top of the wrist (the most common spot), the forearm and sometimes the inside of the elbow. They don't prefer the latter, however, because when the patient bends his arm it tends to dislodge the IV.

Nurses are most adept at putting in IVs, so I knew that if the nurse attending to Max was having a problem it was not due to any lack of ability to do her job. Even so, hospital procedure required her to call in a senior nurse to see if she would have any better luck; when the new nurse was also unable to get an IV in, a third, even more senior, nurse was recruited. She too had no success.

When the nurses couldn't find an acceptable vein, I ordered a central line IV. This is not something I like to do. A central line means I am putting in an IV catheter that directly connects with the patient's heart. It takes anywhere from fifteen minutes to an hour depending on how easily I can find a central vein. There is an inherent risk involved. I could have chosen the subclavian vein, but that would risk puncturing a lung. That could result in pneumothorax, the induction of air or gas into the lungs. If that happened the patient would have a new problem, one that didn't exist before coming under my care. When a medical professional contributes to a new medical problem for a patient, it's known as iatrogenesis. In other words, it's my fault: I made a sick patient sicker. That's not something ER doctors, or any physicians for that matter, want to have happen.

If you want to put the catheter into the right place, the best way is to use a bedside ultrasound machine. In almost all cases, ultrasound allows you to find the correct spot on the first try. Unfortunately, at the time, I wasn't acquainted thoroughly enough with ultrasound to insert a central line (I since have taken courses to get up to speed on this most helpful technology) and was not ready to use it. I needed to do it the old-fashioned way and the sooner the better. Max's blood pressure was dropping quickly.

I wish I could say that finding one of the veins leading into the heart is a precise art. It's not. It's a combination of anatomical knowledge and guesswork. Using anatomical landmarks that are visible on the skin, you insert the needle carefully. There are all kinds of rules for deciding where to insert. Take, for instance, when you put a central line into the femoral vein, a large vein that drains blood from the leg. First, you feel for the pulsations of the femoral artery, which are usually felt at the midpoint of the groin. Textbooks of anatomy state that the femoral vein is approximately one finger's breadth to the inside of the artery; in other words, it's a finger's breadth closer to the inside of the thigh than the artery is.

There's one big problem with the anatomy books: 50 percent of the time the vein is not where it is supposed to be. It may be more than one finger's breadth away from the artery. Instead of inside, it may be on the outside of the artery. The femoral vein may be underneath the artery. You feel the artery and poke, scrub and cleanse the skin, put sterile drapes all around it and freeze the skin. Then you prepare a large needle with a bevelled end—it's hollow but comes to a fine point that looks like a spear—push the needle all the way in and then pull it all the way back. Hopefully you get this beautiful flush of venous blood that is purplish-red.

Often, you have to poke around blindly—there's no other word for it—and it can often take three or four pokes to find the right spot. The big concern with Max was my fear of hitting an artery in the neck. If you put the catheter of the central line in the artery, you can cause a stroke. It's not something for the faint-hearted. Nor is it something for a loved one to watch. I asked Doris to leave, and briefed my resident on what I was going to do and how I was going to do it.

The first try didn't work. I reinserted the needle. Again, I got no blood back in the syringe. Sometimes, if the patient is in shock you may actually have successfully entered the vein but the shock has caused it to collapse. I had no way of knowing if this was the case with Max. On the third try I succeeded. About thirty minutes after I'd started rooting around for a vein, Max was getting saline, followed by blood, and then octreotide and pantoprazole, in that precious intravenous lifeline.

This kind of moment, this kind of challenge, is what I live for in the ER. I had a patient who desperately needed an IV to be successfully inserted so he could receive medication vital to keeping him alive. It took all my skill and courage to find the vein, considering that I knew a slight mistake could kill or seriously imperil him. At the same time, if I didn't get the line, Max could die of irreversible shock. This is one of the challenges that separate ER doctors from people with mundane jobs. Police officers, firefighters and a few other professionals also encounter those types of moments, although I sense ER doctors have a lot more of them. Depending on what cases come through the door, I could be put in a position several times a shift where my actions mean life or death for a patient. And not just occasionally. Shift after shift after shift.

By this point, the initial blood tests taken when Max arrived started to round out the picture. Max's creatinine, a test that measures kidney function, was sky-high compared with those of his last admission to Mount Sinai. Max had developed hepatorenal syndrome, a condition in which both his liver and kidneys were failing at the same time. This was grave news. When I was a fourth-year medical student on my second month of internal medicine, being well supervised by a senior resident and an eminent kidney specialist, I watched helplessly as a middle-aged woman with advanced liver cirrhosis died of hepatorenal syndrome. She was one of the first patients to die on my watch. I didn't want the same thing to happen to Max.

Max's kidneys were rapidly deteriorating. He needed a liver transplant as soon as possible. Doris said he had seen a transplant specialist and was on a waiting list. I silently wished them well but knew that the wait could be long, too long probably for Max. Unless he received a liver transplant right away he was not going to survive much longer.

Doris again pressed me for the prognosis I felt certain she already knew. "What are his chances?" she asked.

"Unless he gets a transplant soon," I said, "they're not good."

The wait for a liver transplant in Canada is unpredictable. The Canadian Liver Foundation estimates it can range from twenty-four hours to three years. That's a hell of a range. Those with an immediate need are obviously at the top of the list, and Max qualified in that regard, based on my assessment. And he was fairly young, another plus.

There's nothing harder than dealing with dying patients and their loved ones. Anyone who says differently is either lying or repressing their true feelings. No matter how many seminars you've taken on the ways to communicate bad news, it's another matter when you have to face people and tell them they have a terminal illness.

"Don't use euphemisms," Dr. Michael Grodin told *ABC News* in 2008. The director of medical ethics at Boston University School of Public Health, Grodin trains residents on how to tell patients they're dying. He advises his students to say "died" and never "passed away" in situations of emergency room traumas. "You have to use the words 'terminal illness' and explain it's quite serious."

Grodin is also leery about estimating how much longer a person has to live. "It's not [a doctor's] job to take away hope but to try to provide support and be as realistic as possible," he says. "We are notoriously bad at predicting how much time a patient has left. You can obviously say that if someone has metastatic cancer that it's unlikely they're going to live for years. But then again I've seen time and time again patients living much longer [than predicted] or dying much sooner."

Being frank is easier said than done in the ER. I wish every patient with a life-threatening illness arrived several hours *before* their heart needed saving, so we could have an honest chat about what to do should the worst happen.

Not that long ago, I was working at Mount Sinai when paramedics brought in an eighty-seven-year-old woman near death. She lived in a nursing home, where a nurse noticed she was having trouble breathing and called 911. As the paramedics wheeled the woman into the resuscitation room, I could see she was in serious trouble.

"She has a history of congestive heart failure," one of the paramedics said as the ER nurses helped move her onto the gurney.

"I can't breathe," she wheezed, pink froth oozing from her lips. When a patient says she can't breathe, you believe her. Her heart was indeed failing. It's the job of the left ventricle—the main pumping chamber of the heart—to thrust rich, red oxygenated blood fresh from the lungs into the aorta, where it can feed the arteries that nourish the vital organs. As the ventricle fails, blood intended to go forward backs up into the lungs, causing the air passages to fill up with blood. This was compounding my patient's struggle to breathe by making it even harder for her to extract oxygen from each breath.

My eyes took a visual snapshot of her condition. She sat bolt upright on the gurney in an instinctive effort to use gravity to keep the blood that was filling up her lungs to stay down. Her face and neck had a dusky blue colour known as cyanosis, a telltale sign she was asphyxiating. A look of fear and intense concentration told me she knew she was in the fight of her life.

I'd seen that look many times before. I knew her heart was mere moments away from stopping. The RT (respiratory therapist) was near the head of my patient's gurney, setting up a bag valve mask to manually force oxygen into the lungs.

"Let's intubate her," I said to the RT. She nodded in agreement as she broke out the intubation tray. In a microsecond, I made the decision to put my patient on a ventilator to try and buy some time to get the excess fluid off her lungs.

"What's her code status?" a nurse asked. Good question. "Code status" is short for advance directives. You hope that every patient who comes to the ER has a piece of paper or a card that tells us what they or their next of kin would like us to do if their heart stops or they need to be put on a ventilator.

Unfortunately, many patients we see in the ER do not have advance directives or a living will. Or the advance directives they do have are so vague it's uncertain how to apply them in a life-or-death situation. On July 28, 2009, United States President Barack Obama announced publicly that he and First Lady Michelle Obama had living wills. He was the first U.S president in history to do so. It remains to be seen whether moral suasion will encourage more people to make their wishes known.

I looked at my frightened patient, wondering what she wanted me to do. All I could see was a woman who was drowning in her own blood and locked in a mortal struggle to survive.

"We're going to put a tube down your throat to help you breathe," I said as matter-of-factly as I could. "We'll give you some medication to help you relax." I squeezed her shoulder. She nodded as best she could. That would have to do for informed consent.

"Five milligrams of Versed and a hundred of propofol," I said to one of the nurses. My patient's laboured struggle to breathe came to a peaceful end as the sedation took effect. The RT and I laid my patient flat, and I moved into position behind her head to insert a breathing tube.

"Number seven and a half?" the RT asked me, referring to the calibre of the endotracheal tube. I nodded. I opened the curve blade of the laryngoscope, the instrument that helps push the tongue out of the way and illuminates the way to the airway, where I needed to insert the tube.

With my long history of early struggles with intubation, I held my breath as the laryngoscope blade neared the epiglottis. I smiled with relief as the cords came into view. I slid the endotracheal tube through the cords and into the airway with ease.

"Sats are up to 92 percent," said the RT as she secured the tube with tape and connected it to the ventilator. "Sats" refers to oxygen saturation, a measure of how much oxygen is coursing through a patient's arteries. A normal saturation is 96 to 100 percent. The lower the stats fall below 96, the more a person is in trouble. A patient whose saturation drops below 90 probably needs to be put on oxygen. When the sats drop to the mid 80s, the person is getting into serious danger of cardiac arrest.

Patients on ventilators are considered too gravely ill to be admitted to a bed on the general internal medicine floor. My patient would have to go to the intensive care unit. I paged the resident. Within an hour, the patient was admitted to the ICU, her life saved, at least this time.

ER physicians make that kind of decision every day. Dr. John Ross is a staff emergency physician and former head of emergency medicine at Queen Elizabeth II Health Sciences Centre in Halifax, Nova Scotia. On *White Coat, Black Art*, I quizzed him about having to make the terrible decision to put patients on life support without knowing their wishes.

"Do we do the tube in the throat and the pounding on the chest?" Ross asked rhetorically. "Or do we take dad or grandfather and make him really comfortable [without putting him on life support]? The problem with that second option is that it takes me hours. It takes a lot of time to do that. In a busy department, there's a built-in disincentive to do that, because I know that if I take that time the people that are in the waiting room to see me are not going to get in because I'm busy [discussing life-support matters] with that one family. So, many of my colleagues and sometimes me, we'll do all the exciting stuff and go on to our next patient . . . but ultimately then, that [first] patient goes to the ICU and occupies a bed."

Dr. Ross's colleague Jill Lambeth, a veteran ER nurse at QEII Health Sciences Centre who has worked alongside Ross for years, puts it even more succinctly. "It's easier to put somebody on life support and to start all the drugs that we use to bring them somewhat back to life until families or whatever group of friends can maybe recognize that there's not going to be a positive outcome," she said on *White Coat, Black Art*. "But sometimes it's almost like, let's leave it up to somebody else to make the decision—like passing the buck."

Lambeth puts at least part of the blame on patients for failing to sign a living will or another form of advance directive. "Often, perhaps 80 percent of the time, we see patients' families wanting us to pull out all the stops and we're just shaking our heads," she says. "It makes you feel helpless. You don't feel ethically you're doing the right thing. You want to provide comfort, and you want to support the patient and their family. You want them to understand that it is hopeless. But their perspective is that this is their father or their mother or their sister, and they just want them to live at any cost."

Ross says these dilemmas over life and death are having an effect on overcrowded emergency departments like the one he works in. "When I look around my emergency department today, for instance, I see that there are about eight or ten patients that are admitted with no place to go."

Talking to people like John Ross and Jill Lambeth, one might get the sense that all families clamour to have their loved ones pulled back from the brink of death and put on ventilators ad infinitum. Sometimes, it's the exact opposite.

A few years ago, I was on duty at Mount Sinai Hospital when paramedics brought in a sixty-seven-year-old man who had collapsed after complaining of a headache. As he was wheeled into the resuscitation room, I quickly recognized that my patient had all the symptoms of a massive stroke. He was moaning incoherently and was in great distress. Still, I needed to confirm my provisional diagnosis by ordering a CT scan of his head. Trouble was, he was showing signs of swelling inside the brain, likely due to a cerebral hemorrhage. Slowly, the hemorrhage was expanding inside the bony confines of his skull, squeezing what was left of his intact brain. In particular, it was putting pressure on a part of the brain called the medulla oblongata, which enables us to breathe without putting any thought into it.

As with my eighty-seven-year-old patient, I made a quick decision to intubate. I wanted to buy time to stabilize him so we could send him for the CT scan. I placed him on a ventilator as well.

About forty minutes later, he was brought back from the CT room, and my grim suspicions were confirmed. He had a massive intracerebral hemorrhage from which recovery was unfortunately unlikely.

His brother and eldest son had arrived, along with their spouses and children. I gathered the family in a quiet room to explain what had happened. To this point, the family hadn't seen their loved one. When I explained why I had put his father on a ventilator, the son stopped me.

"I wish you hadn't done that," he said in a tone both upset and accusatory. I was perplexed.

The son explained that, as a young man, his father had witnessed his own mother have a subarachnoid hemorrhage caused by a burst aneurysm. The doctors worked heroically to save her life. However, she lived the next fifteen years in a vegetative state.

"My father told us many times that he didn't want the same thing to happen to him," the son explained. The patient's brother immediately corroborated his nephew's account.

Here I was, congratulating myself for doing a slick intubation and stabilizing my patient quickly and—I hate to use the word—efficiently, when all the time, if he could have spoken, he would have said he wanted to be left to die with dignity.

After a long conversation with the family, I was asked by the patient's son to withdraw life support. From the very same bedside at which I had prolonged my patient's life, I now took away the tube and the ventilator sustaining his vital functions. He died moments later, his family gathered around the gurney.

When it comes to talking to patients, the watchword is "informed consent." That's a legal condition whereby patients give consent to treatment (or to no treatment), having been informed of the facts and the implications of saying yes or no. To do so, they have to be free of conditions that affect their ability to comprehend the choices. In practical terms, that means they must be free of dementias like Alzheimer's disease, intoxication with alcohol and other drugs, and mental illness or diseases that might affect the powers of reason.

These days, doctors are taught to be as scrupulously honest as possible about a patient's chance of survival. We're leery of being accused of peddling false hope. I've seen many physicians, in an effort to be honest, go overboard and develop an approach that I perceive as brutal.

In my own hospital, when I've referred an elderly patient to the internal medicine service, I've seen residents barely introduce themselves before asking the patient or the family if the patient has advance directives. Sometimes, when I ask residents from internal medicine or the ICU to see a patient of mine in the ER, they ask by training and by reflex if the patient has a signed "Do Not Resuscitate," or DNR, order, on the chart, even before they get to know the patient or the family.

Don't get me wrong. With my patient who had the cerebral hemorrhage, it would have been very helpful to me and comforting to the patient and his family if I had known his wishes in advance. I see no problem figuring out things in advance. It's just that I also feel it's wrong for a medical practitioner to be unnecessarily blunt and hasty about the subject simply because a patient is ill and needs to consider a decision regarding life support.

When we behave this way, we abandon patients and their families at one of the most difficult times in their lives. If I happen to overhear a resident pressing a family for a DNR, I sometimes sense the same kind of "no haggle" tone I get from car salesmen when I'm looking for a new car.

Counsellors and psychologists believe that residents may be hard-boiled in their approach to families of patients in peril because they've been scarred by the relentless pace of hospital medicine. Experts suggest residents may be suffering from what's known as "compassion fatigue." Also known as secondary traumatic stress disorder, compassion fatigue is a term that refers to a gradual lessening of compassion over time. The term was first attributed to nurses in the 1950s. It's common among people who experience trauma and especially among health care professionals who regularly see patients in traumatic circumstances, especially life-threatening injuries.

If that's the case, the fault may lie with attending physicians who go home to sleep at night, leaving residents on-call to deal with patients and families on the edge between life and death.

Up to now, I've talked a lot about heroic efforts to pull patients back from that very brink, and whether or not we should attempt it. But all too often, when we preoccupy ourselves with those pursuits, we forget that the patient is not only ill but may be quite aware that he's dying.

As a student, I believed that truth is to medicine what a steel girder is to an office tower: solid, hard to bend and impossible to break. Time and experience have taught me that's not always the case. Doctors may shade the truth, or lie by omission, or even outright deceive because we believe that, in some cases, it's better medicine.

"I dare you to find a doctor who hasn't lied to a patient at some point in their career," said Dr. Philip Hébert on *White Coat, Black Art*. Dr. Hébert is the author of *Doing Right: A Practical Guide to Ethics for Medical Trainees and Physicians*. "Lies come in various sorts, don't they? Small lies, big lies. Probably most of us are comfortable with the white lie."

He recalls one patient who was within a month or two of dying. When the patient said he thought he looked healthy and asked for Hébert's opinion, the doctor agreed with him, even though he thought otherwise, which was an obvious lie.

"I kept it to myself because I wasn't prepared to have that conversation that day," Hébert says. "I did it for me . . . but my primary motivation was for him. I thought that the truth wasn't what he wanted to hear. I sensed that he wanted support for his belief that he looked okay."

The patient died soon after. Though it happened years ago, Hébert regrets it to this day.

"It was an opportunity for a conversation that I missed," he says. "If I'd picked up on the fact that I was saying what I said as much for me as for him, I would have said that maybe this was the time to have a conversation with him about impending death . . . a conversation that we often don't have, that we put off."

Hébert talks about the code doctors use to communicate things without actually saying them. For instance, if you get a call from a doctor or a nurse telling you to come to the hospital right away, it probably means a loved one is either dead or near death, with little chance of recovery.

"People sometimes hear what they want to hear," says Hébert. "You can say it in such a way that they know the real message—and you know they know the real message—and yet nobody talks about what the real message is. So patients and their families might participate in the collusion."

It's amazing how much deception goes on in medicine. "There's never any class on 'Deception 101,'" he says. "But truth is to be dispensed like any other drug. To be dispensed if it has good outcomes, and to be withheld if it has bad outcomes, in the physician's mind." He says admonishments like that are as old as Hippocrates.

Hébert acknowledges the tectonic shift in the doctor-patient relationship brought on by the duty to provide informed consent. But he says age has mellowed his zeal for accuracy in truth telling.

"I think as I get older in practice, I tend to be a little more paternalistic, a little bit more protective of my patients," he says, surprising himself as he speaks. "I'm not quite as ready to rush in with the truth. If I think my patients' autonomy is compromised by illness, I want to help them regain their autonomy. The 'soft' kind of paternalism encourages health professionals to use their clinical acumen to decide whether a patient's autonomy is compromised to the extent that they can't handle the whole truth today."

The only possible exception, in Hébert's mind, occurs when a patient is at risk of dying and may not know it.

"A friend of mine who is an anaesthetist was rushing a patient to the operating room," he says. "He'd been in a car accident. He had a lacerated liver and was likely to die. The patient was conscious enough to ask the anaesthetist if he was going to make it."

Hébert says his anaesthetist friend made a split-second decision to assure the patient he'd be all right, even though she believed he would die. Unfortunately, the patient succumbed to his injuries.

"I think if I were the person who was about to probably die, I wouldn't mind that being brought to my attention," says Hébert. "Maybe I could tell someone the fortune is hidden in the third elm tree in the park. There may be some important news you want to pass on. So, you've got to tell patients if things aren't looking too good. I haven't quite figured out what the right script is. But if you don't tell them the truth, then that terrible secret they've held for, say, the past twenty-five years, they can't pass on to somebody else. I think the biggest problem with deception is that we don't give patients the chance to confront the truth, as they have to, at some point."

As hard as it is to talk to patients about their impending mortality, I find it much more heart-wrenching to inform loved ones that a person has died in the ER. Not surprisingly, there's no way to predict how people will react to such news.

When I was early in my career and still working at another hospital, a young female summer student, maybe nineteen, was brought to the ER after being electrocuted on a construction site. She had been operating a piece of equipment that struck a power line. The voltage surge literally cooked every organ in her body, including her heart. She was dead on arrival and nothing could be done to revive her.

I can still see her father and uncle arriving at the ER, a look of cold shock draped all over them. It was up to me to tell them what had happened, and they absorbed it as if being told an item on the news. They didn't say a word, just turned and walked away, numb to the core. I know it wasn't a matter of them being uncaring; this was the way they dealt with it on the spot, in public. Shock can do that to you. There's no "proper" way to respond.

I recall a friend telling me about his fifty-something mother-in-law wanting to return to work the day after her husband suddenly died. "Her relatives were appalled when she said this," he said, "and clucked their disapproval." He, however, knew it was his mother-in-law's way of trying to cope with the sudden upheaval in her life. "She was grasping on to the only stable thing she could think of." She didn't end up going to work, he said, but even if she had, if that's what she needed to do to get through the next day or the one after that, who was he or anyone else to judge her?

I have, of course, also witnessed a reaction to death opposite to the composed response of the summer student's relatives. While certain cultures tend to be stoic, others seem to need to make a loud and very public display of grief. I know these are generalizations, but I have to say they have proven quite accurate, based on my own observations.

One time I had to inform a large group of extended family members that their loved one had died in the ER. It was an unexpected death, as she had not been ill before coming in that night suffering from a heart attack. A couple of her children began to cry and wail; others quickly joined in, and it was soon a hysterical scene with people literally bouncing off the walls and striking themselves. I was taken aback by the public and vocal outpouring of emotions—I am more stoic in nature—but it was not my place to judge how they responded.

It was hard not to be judgmental when I was told about a case that had happened just before I came on duty for a shift. A middle-aged man who was obese had collapsed and been rushed to the ER a few moments after he and a large number of family members had arrived at a professional sporting event. The paramedics accurately diagnosed him as having suffered a heart attack. They advised the rest of the family that the father's condition was grave. His eldest daughter accompanied him to Mount Sinai in the ambulance, but the rest—three adults and two preteens—stayed behind to watch the game.

"Dad was a sports nut and would have wanted them to go ahead and go to the game," she told the ER doctor who was on duty before me. "We saved up forever for the tickets, which we bought from a scalper for a lot of money. The [young] boys had never been to a game before." As the ER team intubated the father and did everything they could to save him—to no avail, unfortunately—the daughter kept in touch with the rest of the clan via cellphone. He died just before I clocked in, which was around the time the game ended. It wasn't long after that the family converged en masse in the ER. By then I was on duty. I heard them crying and displaying the kind of affection their actions seemed, on the surface, to belie. But who was I—or any of the rest of us who, quite frankly, spent some time that night discussing the unusual circumstances of the case—to criticize the family's decision?

"I couldn't have stayed at the game, knowing he might die," a staff member said, a feeling that it's fair to say the majority of us shared.

"Maybe it was the best thing for the young boys," someone else suggested. "It distracted them from what was going on here. Did they really need to be in the ER the whole time their grandfather was dying?" That was a good point too, I thought.

In the end, what did it matter to me (or any of my co-workers) how the family managed the situation? It seemed obvious from their reaction to his death that their love for the deceased was genuine. I'm sure there are others who sit for hours at a dying person's side who don't really love the person but do it for show. Is one reaction right and the other wrong? No way of knowing. Only the people themselves know what is in their hearts. Those of us on the outside have no right to criticize or endorse whatever course of action they take.

Fortunately, we don't deal with a lot of dying patients at Mount Sinai's ER. My chief, Howard Ovens, estimates that, on average, maybe one or two patients die in a week. The vast majority of those deaths are considered expected in that they occur in patients who are elderly or who have advanced cancer and other serious diseases. Still, I have personally worked for months, even a year or two, without a death during one of my shifts.

Not so the ER doctors in some U.S. cities. When Dr. Bruce Campana worked at the Tri-City Medical Center in Oceanside, California (Tri-City refers to Oceanside, Vista and Carlsbad—near San Diego), he was exposed to death on a far more regular basis than I have ever experienced. One case involving an illegal migrant worker and her child has forever haunted him.

The Mexican illegals tended to come to the hospital at night, when there was less of a chance of being nabbed by an immigration officer. They came in families, Campana says, and were invariably polite and well behaved. The hospital treated whoever showed up.

The evening in question a young mother ran into the ER, bypassing the triage nurse. Campana happened to be in her path, and she handed him a child who was perhaps eighteen months to two years old. "As soon as she handed me the child I could feel the child's skin; it was cold," he says. The mother didn't speak English, but the look on her face made it clear she was greatly concerned. "I looked down and the child was not breathing. I took the child to the resuscitation bay. Holy shit, for the first time in my life I would be doing mouth-to-mouth resuscitation. I had vowed never to do mouth-to-mouth unless it was a supermodel, and I would now break my vow . . . on this cold dead child. As I did, the child's cold vomit came into my mouth. I started CPR and bagging [administering an IV] as the team arrived." The team worked for about twenty minutes, trying everything to save the child even though they knew there was no point. The child was dead. The cause was probably dehydration as a result of chronic diarrhea.

Campana's momentary aversion to mouth-to-mouth was understandable. It was the late 1980s, and some physicians were rightly concerned about catching HIV by ingesting saliva. More than that, as emergency physicians, we aren't first responders, which means we seldom do mouth-to-mouth. I can remember vividly a time when I was escorting a stretcher-bound patient who suffered an unanticipated cardiac arrest during which he aspirated food. His mouth was covered in vomitus. I knew it was going to take a precious couple of minutes to find an oropharyngeal airway to insert into the patient's mouth and to start bag-ventilating him. I allowed myself to feel revolted for an instant, then started mouth-to-mouth. The man survived. When I had a free moment, I ducked into a bathroom and brushed my teeth for about fifteen minutes.

Campana says a dying child has a way of galvanizing people in the ER to leave their comfort zone. "You'll see people move that you haven't seen move before. Some people don't seem to be scared or [motivated to move quickly] by any event in emergency. But when a child comes in and is dying, you will see these people have a change of heart. It was nurses that you might consider lazy. It was porters that always seemed to be on break and never seemed to be doing anything. The doc who was going to leave at midnight and is by your side and helping out. A change in heart that takes exceptional circumstances to bring about."

The mother had been present during the desperate last-ditch resuscitation attempt because everyone was so focused on trying to help the child they didn't think to ask her to leave. "I personally don't have a problem with families in the resuscitation room," says Campana. "I think it is good for them to see we are doing everything [possible]. Although I hate the term, it gives them some closure. At a time when so much is being taken from them, giving them that is the least health professionals can do."

If by some miracle they'd gotten a pulse for the child, Campana thinks it would probably not have been the best outcome, for the lack of oxygen to the brain would have caused irreparable damage. Although children have been known to make miraculous recoveries, the odds of that happening are incredibly small, and in this case virtually impossible. For adults, until quite recently, resuscitation following a prolonged period of oxygen deprivation was something few physicians would have wanted to happen. "Most people don't understand that. Adults come back brain damaged and dysfunctional. You have a family who is initially grateful and then two months, six months, a year down the road they're asking: 'Why did you bring this person back? Why didn't you bring them back completely? Why did you just bring part of them back?' It isn't fair to anybody—the patient, the family or the system, if you will."

But none of this made any difference to that little child and its mother so many years ago. Campana remembers the look on her face when she knew there was no hope for her child. It was "a pain that I can only imagine as a parent and that I don't ever want to feel. As a third party there is nothing to compare to the utter devastation of [being with] a parent that has lost a child. To see the walls crumble. All the metaphors you want to use. It is a horrible thing to see [but at the same time] what an honour to be there. What an obligation to do what we do, whether it's the work on the patient or telling [the news] to the parent. They are going to remember that we handled their child gently, put our hand on their child, or we had tears in our eyes. They are going to remember that their entire life, not how quickly we intubated."

As Campana reflects back on that night, he sees it in a light that might seem surprising. "Terrible to say, but it is thrilling to be involved in a life-and-death situation and to be pivotal in that. It is a fundamental concept for any emergency physician. It sounds terrible to say 'thrilling,' as if I'm happy and glad, but I am not. Your heart races and your mind is sharp. It is part of why we do. I am not sure I can articulate it better than that."

When asked how the mother and the rest of her family reacted to the death, Campana nervously makes a generalization. "Pardon me if I make a broad and probably a false statement: Mexicans grieve honestly. Mexican families cried and were upset and did what I think they are supposed to do. They hurt and it showed and you felt for them. There are families I have seen where there are bizarre reactions ranging from apparent indifference to shows, as if they clearly wanted a hidden camera to be there to see the drama as they punched the wall and did all the other things you see on TV. That leaves you with a bad taste in your mouth."

Dr. Peter Rosen, Campana's mentor and one of the pioneers of emergency medicine, used to tell a story about taking care of a young man who died in a car crash. Rosen phoned the father and told him the news.

"You need to come down, your son has been badly hurt in a car crash," Rosen said.

"Do I have to come now?" the father asked.

"Yes, right away."

"Is he dead?"

"I am sorry to tell you that he is."

"Then I don't have to come now, do I?" the father said.

Says Campana: "Rosen would tell this story, shaking his head, as one extreme example of the human experience of telling people."

An emergency ward, Campana says, is a "minefield," and no matter how carefully you negotiate your way through such a place, disasters such as death invariably occur. "Better learn soon in your career: you can do things right and people can die. You can obey all the rules and be up to date on your literature and treatment and, goddamn it, some people just die. To form a human bond and have that person die in front of you is one of the most wrenching experiences a doctor can have."

One of the mines we have to deal with in the ER involves patients who have done something terrible to others. Drunk drivers are among the most common to fall into this category.

For more than twenty years, Bruce Campana has been going to high schools to talk about the need to drive safely. Inevitably a student asks him to tell his worst-ever car crash story. He has no trouble recalling it.

Paramedics, accompanied by the police, brought in a forty-something man who had been in a horrific accident that night. He had been alone in his car when a drunk driver struck right where he was sitting. The paramedics had performed CPR on the victim, attached an IV and then intubated him. When Campana examined the man he found no pulse.

"I decided to open up his chest, not knowing what else I could do," says Campana. "I poured sterilizing agent all over his chest and cut it open with a scalpel. I go in to reach for his heart and his heart wasn't there. His heart had been ripped free and thrown to the right side of his chest, and there was a lake of blood. He was clearly dead. We stopped. I said what I always say: 'Sorry, everybody, the time is such and such.' Everybody cleaned up because everybody was a mess. There was nothing else to do."

Although greatly disturbed by what he had just experienced, Campana, like any ER doctor, had to move on to his next patient. As he picked up the chart, one of the paramedics told him the patient was the driver of the other car.

"The guy was a drunk, an obnoxious forty- or fifty-year-old male," he says. "He was bruised and there were cuts, one on his head. It wasn't as if his limbs were splayed and there was blood oozing out of him. I couldn't stop myself. I said, 'Do you know you killed that man?' The guy said, 'Fuck him. Just fix my head.' I became somewhat unprofessional. For the only time in my life I forgot to use a local anaesthetic when I was fixing his cut. I was cleaning it quite thoroughly, and you have to be quite rough to do that. He objected to that. I didn't respond to his objections. He got up off the bed, pushed me, I pushed back. [There was] a shouting match between us. The police separated us and took him away. I remember thinking I wanted to kill him. I wanted him to die. I didn't do anything, of course. I remember hating him more than any other person I'd ever met."

I had a similar experience more than twenty years ago. A drunk driver had hit a car carrying two elderly couples, one of them the parents of Arlene Perly-Rae, the wife of Liberal MP and former Ontario premier Bob Rae. Three died instantly and the fourth succumbed to his injuries a few hours later at Sunnybrook Health Sciences Centre. As so often happens, the driver of the other vehicle survived. He had fairly minor scrapes and bruises and was brought to York Central Hospital to be patched up.

No matter what had happened to these innocent people, and the endless pain brought into the lives of their loved ones, you have to treat the man as a patient and not a criminal. At the same time, in cases such as these you might be a little slower to administer a pain-killer or you might shove a catheter in a little harder than is required. I have fantasized about doing both at times. This particular person had so few injuries that all I could do was clean him up, knowing at least that a pair of handcuffs was waiting for him once I had completed my work.

4:02 A.M.

Fortunately, we didn't have to deal with the death of Max that night. As I finished up in the resuscitation room, I wondered if I should talk to Doris about what I felt certain was the ultimate cause of her husband's problems. Just before we had begun to work on Max I reminded the nurses, and myself, to be especially careful about being in contact with Max's blood. "Do any of you have any cuts?" I asked. No one did. "If you get cut in any way at any time, you have to get the cut covered completely right away. Don't take any chances. And make sure your surgical gloves have no nicks in them."

I suspected that Max was HIV positive, but I didn't know for sure. It wasn't on his chart and Doris hadn't said anything. There weren't many other reasons why someone his age would have all these medical problems. It was an educated guess on my part but nothing more than that. Did she know or sense it? Did I have an obligation to say something to her?

As I debated what to do, Doris resolved my dilemma. "I'm going to go out for a while," she said to me quietly. "Max has a friend, a very dear friend, who's going to come in and see him. I called him because I'm worried that Max won't make it. Please make sure he is allowed to spend time with him." I said that I would.

Doris then took her things and headed outside. Max was lucky,

I thought. She was a fine woman who loved him enough to allow his "friend" a chance to say goodbye. I'm not sure how many other wives would have done the same.

Max survived that night and was transferred to the ICU in the wee hours of the morning. They discharged him a few days later so he could go home to die in peace and with dignity, which he did—of overwhelming liver failure—a few weeks later. I have no way of knowing, but I imagine that both Doris and his friend were by his side. I hope so.

Although there was nothing I could have done to save Max, like every patient who dies, he had an impact on me. The deaths that send the most shivers through a physician involve patients you have sent home in the belief that they no longer need your care—and then a colleague or, worse, a superior, later utters the three words you never want to hear: "Do you remember . . . ?" They are invariably followed by bad news.

When I was a first-year resident in internal medicine at Sunnybrook Health Sciences Centre, I saw a very elderly woman who came to the ER complaining of shortness of breath. I read on her medical chart that she had a history of heart problems.

She had congestive heart failure—her lungs were filling up with water—which meant her heart wasn't pumping blood out efficiently enough. The blood was backing up into her lungs, causing a condition known as pulmonary edema. The backed-up blood reduced the ability of the lungs to exchange carbon dioxide for oxygen. If not treated properly, she would experience respiratory failure.

These days we would put the patient on BiPAP, which stands for bi-level positive airway pressure ventilation. It's a breathing apparatus developed in the 1990s that helps people get more air into their lungs. Basically, it's a large plastic mask that fits over the mouth and forces oxygen under pressure into the lungs. These days, as a last resort, we often intubate a patient and use a ventilator to force oxygen into the lungs, using a mild form of pressure. Back in the early 1980s, when I saw this patient, we mainly gave diuretics, which caused the kidneys to excrete water and sodium, thus reducing the fluid buildup in the lungs. We still give diuretics.

After administering this treatment I ordered some blood tests, which didn't disclose anything to be concerned about. I assessed the woman to be stable and sent her home. Just before doing so, I asked a nurse for her opinion. Being a new doctor, I was a little nervous and wanted a second assessment. I didn't say this to the nurse, but there was a little voice in the back of my head that wasn't 100 percent sure if I was right to release the woman. "I think she'll be okay," the nurse said, which made me feel better.

A few hours later I was about to leave for the day when I heard those three horrible words. "Do you remember . . . the woman you sent home earlier? She's back and she's *in extremis*." This meant she was near death. She had collapsed at home from a heart attack that likely had been smouldering for some time. A heart attack I had missed. Never mind that it hadn't shown up on her electrocardiogram, or that blood tests in those days were nowhere near as sophisticated as they are today. The woman was in her late eighties and was obviously a candidate for a fatal heart attack, especially considering she had had some previous scares. It's easy to say she was living on borrowed time. But perhaps if I had done something differently she would have enjoyed an even longer life. To this day I don't know if I should have discovered it. All I know is that I didn't, and ten days later she was dead. In my heart I still think I blew it by sending her home. Why? Because of that voice in my head, one that as a green doctor I didn't listen to.

It's a funny thing, but I remember her name as if I'd treated her yesterday. I don't often remember the names of the patients I've saved. I almost always remember the names of the ones I've lost.

A wise friend and colleague, now unfortunately passed away, was a well-respected urologist in Hamilton, Ontario. He once told me good judgment comes from experience and experience comes from bad judgment, and I believe it. Since those early cases I've always tried to learn from my mistakes as much as from my triumphs. I was green then; I don't know what colour I am now. What I do know is that when that little voice in my head says something is wrong, I go into red alert. I err on the side of caution, a strategy that's worked well for me.

The truth is, I'd do just about anything not to hear those three awful words ever again.

CHAPTER NINE

LOOKING FOR LOVE
IN ALL THE WRONG PLACES

4:15 A.M.

My next patient was cuddling with her girlfriend on a gurney marooned in the hall near my office. She was in her late twenties and had come in several hours earlier all freaked out after having taken psilocybin mushrooms, known on the street as magic mushrooms or just plain "shrooms." These are naturally occurring fungi that contain the psychedelic compounds psilocybin and psilocin, whose effects can be similar to those found in LSD.

Brenda had eaten a quantity of mushrooms together with her partner, Melinda. As so often happens, one of them had a more intense reaction than the other. When Brenda first arrived at the ER she was terrified she was going crazy, according to the triage nurse's notes. The nurse had asked me, in passing, if she could give Brenda a couple of Ativan tablets to calm her down, which I thought was a good idea. The mild sedatives soon took effect and helped Brenda get through the worst part of her trip. I just needed to check her over before letting her go home.

I came up behind the women and noticed them spooning underneath a thin hospital blanket. They were facing the wall and didn't see me approach. There was nothing inappropriate about their behaviour, although it was the first time I had seen a couple sharing a bed in the hallway. I coughed to get their attention and introduced myself. They both sat up, and Melinda hopped off the gurney to let me deal directly with Brenda.

"How are you doing now?" I asked.

"Better. I was really scared before," Brenda said. "I thought I was losing my mind. I had no idea how bad an overdose was."

I explained that it's difficult to overdose on mushrooms. "You had an intense reaction to them but, as I think the triage nurse told you, it would go away with time."

Melinda chirped in that she had given the same information to Brenda. "I told her we didn't need to come here," she said. "I'm sorry for wasting your time."

I told her never to worry about wasting my time. In my experience, coming to the ER only looks like a waste of time in retrospect. I chatted with both of them for a bit longer to see if there were any other issues that might need to be addressed, but nothing arose. I could have lectured them on the dangers of drug abuse, but I didn't see the point. Whether they continued to use mushrooms or any other drug was up to them.

"You won't tell the police, will you?" Brenda asked. "I have a job and—"

I told her it wasn't our business whether she had taken drugs. "You can go home now if you want."

As they prepared to leave I stopped to think about them. Their apparent willingness to show affection to each other in such a public place made me smile. Who was I to them? Although they had paid attention to what I had to say as a doctor, beyond that I didn't exist. They were totally enraptured with each other, perhaps still in the early throes of love, which is probably what made them stand out to me.

Thanks to the rampant sexual shenanigans on TV shows like *Grey's Anatomy,* and to many a porn film in which busty and lusty nurses jump the bones of hospital patients, some members of the public think the medical workplace is a sexual hotbed. Sorry to burst that balloon, but the truth is that very little sex or romance takes place in hospitals, especially in the ER ward.

Oh sure, it happens from time to time. But the relationships tend to be pretty quick to start and just as quick to end. Not only that, but the lovers tend to be quite discreet. Not too many years ago, I was the last person in the ER to know that a colleague of mine was dating one of the nurses. But that was one fling. Bottom line, it doesn't happen very often. We're too damn busy and too damn tired. Nonetheless, romance can and does blossom among colleagues—is there a workplace where that doesn't happen?—and on rare occasions between doctors and patients.

The latter is a subject of considerable ethical debate. Before delving into it, I have a confession to make. More than twenty years ago and long before I married Tamara, I briefly dated a patient I'd treated on one occasion in the ER. To stay within boundaries of ethical behaviour, I made certain I never again acted as her physician. We went out two or three times, after which I decided that it didn't feel right dating her.

Whenever I hear patients talk about how cute or sexy their doctor is it makes me uncomfortable. True, it makes me wonder if a patient ever thought that about me. It also reminds me that patients are free to talk about and act on their desires. Not so health professionals, who have strict policies to keep them from crossing the line. Boundaries are what safeguard patients and their caregivers from the instant formalized intimacy that happens on the examination table and on the psychiatrist's couch.

When people think about boundaries, they tend to think about dating and sex. But boundaries aren't only about intimate physical contact. You give your physiotherapist a gift that's too generous or too personal. Or you get a hug from your doctor that lasts a few seconds too long and leaves you feeling a bit disturbed. Or you offer to build a deck for the ER nurse who helped pull you through.

Until now, you probably haven't given the rules a moment's thought. But health professionals think about them all the time. That's because boundaries are part of every contact we have with every patient, and because the price of crossing them—possibly losing your licence to practise and being shamed in public—is so great.

Health professionals, be they MDs, nurses, massage therapists and even paramedics, have the power to ask you the most personal questions and to touch you in the most intimate places. They should never seek sexual gratification in an encounter with a patient in return.

Still, some of us cross the line. Sex between doctors and patients does happen. Older studies suggest between 7 and 13 percent of physicians have had sexual or erotic contact with patients at least once in their careers. And it's not just physicians who cross the line. In one study, psychologists, chiropractors and counsellors were found to have had even higher rates of sexual misconduct than MDs.

These days, physicians who have sex with current or recent patients are often thought to be sociopaths—predators who go into medicine to prey on patients and to take advantage of the power they have over them. These doctors are considered the likeliest to reoffend.

Others who cross the line have low self-esteem. Their marriages may be failing, and work is the only place where they feel successful. If a patient idolizes a doctor, then the table may be set for a relationship. But such MDs usually feel guilty about what they've done, and seldom do it again.

To be brutally honest, that just about sized me up on that night shift more than twenty years ago.

Hard to believe, but not that long ago when a new MD set up shop in a one-doctor town, it was fairly common for the physician to find a willing marriage partner among his or her patients. In those days, many health professionals crossed the line because they didn't know the line existed. Today, provincial colleges and state boards of medicine have fairly precise rules regarding the conduct between a health professional and a patient. The rules of proper conduct are taught in med school and in residency. But back when I had my brief relationship, the topic of boundaries between doctor and patient was awash in a bath of unhealthy shame. In medical school, my mentors avoided the subject completely. By inference, it was certainly clear that having sex with a current patient was a "no-fly zone," so to speak. But beyond that, the rules were less black and white than grey. In large part that was because guilt and shame kept patients and health professionals from talking about the subject.

All that changed in Ontario in January 1991, when the provincial College of Physicians and Surgeons appointed lawyer Marilou McPhedran to head its independent Task Force on Sexual Abuse of Patients. The task force heard from patients who had been abused repeatedly by their physician. Some accounts were recent; others went back decades. Many spoke for the first time of their experiences at the hands of health professionals. What was striking was how many people developed lifelong afflictions like depression and substance abuse as a result.

The task force made sixty recommendations designed to protect patients from predatory physicians; many, though not all, were implemented by the college. In an article published in 1992 in the *Canadian Medical Association Journal,* McPhedran said she was stung by criticism she had received from individual physicians and from organizations like the Ontario Medical Association. "Look, guys," McPhedran told representatives of the OMA, "why are you evading the issue? You're wrong on this—wrong legally, medically, socially and morally."

Among McPhedran's many recommendations was a zero-tolerance policy on sex between doctors and patients. "Due to the position of power the physician brings to the doctor-patient relationship, there are NO circumstances—NONE—in which sexual activity between a physician and a patient is acceptable," she wrote in her final report. "Sexual activity between a patient and a doctor ALWAYS represents sexual abuse, regardless of what rationalization or belief system the doctor chooses to use to excuse it. Doctors need to recognize that they have power and status, and that there may be times when a patient will test the boundaries between them. It is ALWAYS the doctor's responsibility to know what is appropriate and never to cross the line into sexual activity." The college agreed, and a zero-tolerance policy was adopted.

Nowadays, the rules vary among provinces. But we can make some generalizations. For instance, as I've mentioned, it is *verboten* for health professionals to date patients for whom they provide ongoing medical or psychiatric care. That's an easy, black-and-white sort of rule.

From there, it gets murkier. The people who license and monitor health professionals aren't quite so sure what the rules are between health professionals and ex-patients. Some jurisdictions slap a mandatory cooling-off period from the time the doctor–patient relationship concluded until a romantic one can take its place. The duration of the cooling-off period varies with the jurisdiction. The College of Physicians and Surgeons of Ontario has ruled that psychiatrists as well as family physicians engaged primarily in psychotherapy can never date ex-patients.

I suspect there's a much larger group of health professionals who, like me, have asked patients out after providing episodic care— for instance, doctors who work in emergency departments and walk-in clinics—where you see a patient one time only. Some think the rules prohibiting such contact shouldn't apply to them.

Dr. Bruce Campana is one of them. It's one thing to question the boundaries. It's quite another to do so in public. Few doctors, other than those who end up being reported to the college, will admit to having gone out with a patient. I am one of the exceptions. Not surprisingly, the candid Campana is another.

When he was a young ER resident many years ago, one of his rotations was in orthopaedic surgery. That's where the ER doctors send patients with fractured or broken bones.

One night in 1985 an attractive young woman came in with a minor fracture. Campana liked her, and he flirted with her in a mild fashion. She had to return in a few weeks to have her cast removed, and he was still on his orthopaedic rotation. The woman was the last patient of the day. "I thought she was never going to come into my room," Campana said on *White Coat, Black Art*. After taking care of her medical needs he asked her out. To his delight she accepted.

They went to lunch, which Campana describes as being "like a Disney movie. Birds were singing to us. It was spring and the snow was melting. We went to some restaurant. They fussed over us and gave us free dessert. A patient came up in the middle of lunch [and said], 'Oh doctor, you saved my life.' One of those dates you dream about. Incredible. We had so much in common. I liked hiking. She liked hiking. I liked scuba diving. She liked scuba diving. I liked skiing. She liked skiing. I liked women. She liked women. Perhaps more, actually."

The relationship did not progress. "That was a deal breaker," he says. "It was actually a heartbreaker for me."

In going on the date Campana had rationalized that although it was wrong to ask somebody out while you were taking care of her, it was okay to do so afterwards. The abrupt end to his idealized romance seemed to be a warning that his rationalization was just that.

"You always have that twinge in your stomach [that it's wrong] but . . . it starts to get a little bit Bill Clintonesque, doesn't it?" he says. "I didn't have 'relations with that woman' during the period of care. That was my rationalization. I thought this was okay. Frankly, I am not entirely sure that that's wrong. I have trouble with the edict that a doctor can *never* ask a patient out. Now, I don't have trouble with the idea that a physician in an ongoing professional relationship with a patient shouldn't ask somebody out. I don't think a family doctor can ask out a patient. [But] an emergency physician who takes care of a patient once and concludes that care, is it so wrong to ask out a patient when the care is completed?"

I'm not sure there's anything wrong with dating a patient you treated for a minor ailment for a few minutes in the ER if there's a cooling-off period. A year perhaps? Is there still some imbalanced power relationship in play after that amount of time has passed, especially if the initial encounter was not emotionally charged? If the ER doctor had saved the person's life, I can understand that would change the dynamic, yet is it valid to have rules that slip and slide along some kind of care scale? I accept that it was wrong to arrange a date in the ER, as both Campana and I did, as the circumstances probably made us more attractive to the patients, and made them more vulnerable to our advances (although in my case I had not directly initiated our date). But if I had run into the woman months later at a party and from that interaction begun an affair, was I still in a potentially abusive/exploitative position just because I had once repaired a cut?

I see some grey area in the scenarios involving Campana and myself. But there's no question in my mind, and I think among the vast majority of health professionals, that there's a lifetime zero-tolerance policy if any form of therapy or counselling is involved.

In 1998 Canadian writer R.M. Vaughan had an affair with his male psychiatrist. As he recounted on *White Coat, Black Art,* and as he chronicled in his book *Troubled* (published in 2008), Vaughan said he told his doctor one day that he loved him, which often happens in therapy. Instead of discussing Vaughan's infatuation—it's called erotic transference—objectively as part of the treatment, his psychiatrist asked him out to dinner. That night Vaughan went back to the man's house and they had sex. The psychiatrist showered him with gifts, wrote him poetry and asked him to move in. Vaughan was soon spending half the week in the man's home. "If I had met someone in a normal circumstance . . . I would say this was too fast," he says. But he was smitten. "This person knew everything about me and decided I was good enough for him. That is an incredibly powerful way to seduce someone."

A few weeks later the psychiatrist ended it, which plunged Vaughan into a deep depression. "I was in my mid-thirties, and like a lot of people in their mid-thirties, I was lost in my own career, lost in my own progress as an artist, living on next to nothing," Vaughan says. "I had a series of failed relationships, and I sought psychotherapy to unravel my own feelings of failure and my inability to sense accomplishment when it did happen, and why I couldn't connect with other men. That became a primary focus of our therapeutic sessions, [which] was him attempting to teach me to connect with potential romantic partners. I now see that as the first step in his predation."

Among the troubling allegations made by Vaughan was that his psychiatrist constantly put down any of the men Vaughan talked about in their therapy sessions. "Every man I discussed in his office that I had met, had gone on a date with, or was interested in was wrong for me. All my romantic options were worn down by him," he says. "In my feeble state, and it was a kind of a feeble state at the time, one begins to grasp for ropes in the water, and when I reached that moment in therapy that so many patients do, I was in love with the doctor. Instead of him saying, 'No, you're not. This is a stage,' that is when things started."

Vaughan admits he knew what he was doing was wrong. He sought advice from friends, who were divided in their responses. Half told him to walk away from the affair, but the other half encouraged him. "I was at a turning point in my life, and every decision I made was incredibly important, and I was shaping my narrative from the therapeutic line I was being fed. If I had decided not to engage in a romantic relationship with him I would have been not fulfilling some destined role."

The affair came to a close the same way it began, Vaughan says: "Impulsive on his side. I thought I was in love with him. I was beginning a life journey with another person, and within a matter of six to eight weeks he said, 'I don't feel the same way anymore. It's over, and please don't tell anyone.'"

A person in therapy is typically in a heightened emotional state, which makes the ban on relationships with patients so important. "I had a nervous breakdown. I almost killed myself," says Vaughan. "[I was] suffering from massive panic attacks. My rage and hurt were just flying all over the place like this exploded person where the bits of me were everywhere. Finally what happened, people in my life and my GP said, 'What is going on with you? You're a mess.'"

Hearing Vaughan's account made me reflect upon my own brief encounter with a patient following a single treatment in the ER, which happened long before the Independent Task Force on Sexual Abuse of Patients in Ontario. What I did was not in violation of any guidelines at the time. The most recent Ontario College guidelines, published in December 2008, state that "...if a physician saw a patient on one or two occasions to provide routine clinical care, it may not be inappropriate to have a sexual relationship with the former patient within a short time following the end of the physician–patient relationship." That may be the College's view. However, it's something I didn't feel right about twenty years ago and something I never did again.

Dr. Jeff Blackmer, the director of the Canadian Medical Association's Office for Ethics, says he gets constant calls from doctors seeking advice on whether they've crossed the line. Although he agrees that in the past provincial colleges erred too often on the side of the doctors, he now thinks it is probably more the other way around. "There are very few examples recently where you can point to [taking the doctor's side]," he says. "We have examples the other way quite often where a regulatory body will set a penalty or will set a revocation of licence and that will be appealed to the courts. The courts have sometimes said, 'Perhaps in this situation the regulators went too far in protecting the public. The physician did not get due process, wasn't within the guidelines.' The profession at large feels that the college is very strict in terms of enforcing its guidelines. There certainly is no feeling in the profession that there is leniency and self-protectionism."

Like many other jurisdictions nowadays, the College of Physicians and Surgeons of Ontario has on its books a rule that prohibits dating between a doctor and a patient for life if the treatment involved psychotherapy of any kind. A physician convicted of doing that will have his or her licence revoked. That said, the College leaves open the possibility of redemption. A doctor convicted of sexual misconduct can apply to return to practice. To protect public safety, the reinstated physician must agree to specific terms and conditions. Usually they include working on a team with other therapists and never seeing patients without at least one other employee present.

Beyond sex, it may surprise you just how blurred the line between what is okay and what is prohibited can be in practice. Consider something as essential in health care as touching a patient.

"Touch is extremely challenging for physicians because touching patients in intimate ways is an important part of our work," Dr. Barbara Lent, a family physician in London, Ontario, told me on *White Coat, Black Art*. Dr. Lent teaches a course on boundaries for the Ontario College of Physicians and Surgeons. "Touching patients who have just told you a sad story often can be a helpful thing in acknowledging to the patient the impact of that story, acknowledging their distress, acknowledging that you want to help them work through some of their difficulties. But there are times when the touch doesn't necessarily have a simple clinical value."

Lent cites examples of the latter as touching patients on the knee or the thigh, which could be interpreted, whether accurately or not, by some as a sign the physician "wants to develop some kind of special personal relationship" with the patient. She believes doctors have to be trained to know how to communicate that a touch is not that type of signal.

Most doctors, Lent agrees, have probably crossed a boundary line to one degree or another at some time in their careers. "We've probably told people stories about our own lives, shared things.

We've certainly accepted gifts or gone out of our way for particular people who are having some difficulty. I can think of times when I've driven patients places. [We need to] make sure that when we do it we're doing it to meet the patient's needs and not because we're interested in getting more involved in this patient's personal life. And that we're not doing it so this patient is going to think we're just this exceptional, out-of-the-world health-care provider."

"The patient is always blameless because the patient is the patient," says Dr. Gail Robinson, a Toronto psychiatrist and an expert on boundary issues, "especially when the patient comes to see a psychiatrist. Maybe one of their problems is that they use seductive methods in order to engage in relationships. The fact is that the patient's obligation is not to analyze his or her behaviour and understand all the risk, and know about transference and any of those things. It is the doctor who is trained to recognize that."

Matters of transference and boundaries aside, it's impossible to eliminate the natural responses most, if not all, of us have to being in the presence of someone we consider gorgeous. In those instances, I find it best to focus on the clinical problem at hand. But in the presence of bounteous beauty, it can sometimes be difficult. I guess that's what makes us human.

I recall one time when a very famous American TV and movie star showed up at Mount Sinai with a kidney stone. She was an exceptionally beautiful woman. It was hilarious to watch as every red-blooded male doctor, myself included, found a way to catch a glimpse of her. She handled the attention with grace and impressed all of us with her sweet disposition and positive outlook.

Doctors are not monks who have signed an oath of celibacy. My colleagues and I notice patients who are attractive and radiate sex appeal. Since that day more than twenty years ago when I crossed the line, I've chatted socially with patients and on rare occasions have even flirted with them. But I've stayed on the doctor side of the boundary. That's because I can't bear the thought of taking advantage of anyone, especially the people I'm supposed to take care of.

As I passed the stretcher where Brenda and Melinda had been snuggling in the hallway, I smiled at the memory of my brief encounter with the young lovebirds. I needed that little mental boost because it was the point in the night shift when I often started to feel tired and cranky. The best antidote was a demanding case. As I saw my resident approaching I hoped she had just that.

CHAPTER TEN

A CRY FOR HELP

4:32 A.M.

Juan was a fifty-nine-year-old white male who had been brought in by paramedics about seven hours earlier after passing out drunk in a bar. He had a few scrapes on his face and hands from the fall but nothing serious, so the resident let him sleep it off—it was im- possible to communicate with him until he sobered up—before she cleaned him up and took down his history.

About an hour after my resident had seen Juan, I had time to assess him. Thorough as always, the resident briefed me on what she had learned.

Juan had been married, but the marriage had ended several years earlier. The all-day drinking binge that landed him in the ER was the result of his girlfriend ending their relationship, a decision that had caught him entirely off guard. Juan was overweight with a large belly, but otherwise had no obvious health problems, at least any he was willing to tell us about. He had been laid off from a long-standing job when he turned fifty and had been doing contract work ever since. This new arrangement had actually turned out to be better for him financially until recently, when the economy took a downturn. He had lost some clients and wasn't sure he would get them back. The resident had also been able to find out that Juan lived alone and had lost touch with his extended family.

"He said the combination of everything had triggered tonight's drinking bout," the resident said. "He was depressed and drowned himself in ethanol."

"How much of a drinker is he?"

"He says it depends," she said. "He didn't want to talk much. It was hard to get even this amount out of him."

"Do you think he's suicidal?" I asked. I remembered something Truman Capote said, that alcoholism—a subject he knew only too well and that was the cause of his death—was "a coward's suicide." I think there's a lot of truth in that. Men drinking themselves to death—and by far the vast majority we see in the ER are males—is something all of us witness far too often.

"I asked him that directly," she said.

An impressive response. Some residents are afraid to raise the topic with patients. I praised her gumption.

"He said he was okay. Just feeling down from everything. And I can't really blame him. He has a lot on his plate. I said we could send him over to the psychiatric facility if he wanted. Just so they could make sure he was all right. He said he didn't want to go."

"Did you believe him?"

"Yeah, I did," she said. "He wants to go home, and I think we should let him."

My resident's answer hung in the air between us for a moment. In my twenty-five-plus years of emergency medicine, I figure I've seen at least a thousand (if not more) patients who've said they wanted to kill themselves. Very few really meant it, and even fewer attempted suicide in ways that were potentially lethal. Most took a handful of sleeping tablets or over-the-counter pills like Tylenol. Some made a half-hearted attempt to cut their wrists, breaching the skin but somehow never getting anywhere near a major artery or vein, which, if severed, could cause them to bleed to death.

The World Health Organization estimates that every year about one million people commit suicide. The number looks impressive, but that's worldwide. In Canada, each year fewer than 4,000 kill themselves. The vast majority of suicide attempts are non-lethal. Psychiatrists refer to them as suicidal "gestures" or cries for help. Studies show that for every person who commits suicide, forty attempt it. With those odds, an ER physician can go long stretches without seeing a patient who is at high risk of actually doing it.

"I've certainly encountered the patients that we're not worried about," Dr. Bruce Campana said on *White Coat, Black Art*. "I don't mean to be 'gender insensitive' here, but I'm talking about the teenage girl who takes two Ativans and phones her boyfriend and says, 'I've taken an overdose.' And then the boyfriend rushes her to hospital. There's a great deal of drama, and the nurses are rolling their eyes, and the doctors are rolling their eyes. And we [see them] and send them home. Those are the kinds of patients we don't worry about.

"This is usually someone who is quite dependent and quite whiny. They really have no intention of harming themselves, but they have such primitive coping mechanisms that they really don't know what else to do. So they phone 911 and say they intend to kill themselves because that worked the last time. 'I got a sandwich, I got a warm blanket, and I got some attention.'

"Most of them are looking for attention. They're annoying to the staff. You look through their chart and they have twenty-three prior visits to the emergency department for suicidal ideation. The truth is, probably that person is not a big risk."

The operative word is *probably*. You never know for sure. The challenge for ER physicians and psychiatrists is to figure out who means business and to get them help before they succeed. But years and years of seeing people who don't mean it can dull your ability to pick out the ones who do.

Campana believes that ER physicians don't see that many patients who are truly determined to commit suicide because these people kill themselves before they can be brought to the ER. "It's not very hard to kill yourself," he says.

There are numerous studies with varying results, but they all conclude that males are far more likely to take their own lives than females. According to a 1999 study conducted by Washington University Medical School, 75 percent of the 30,000 Americans who kill themselves each year are male. I've seen other studies that place the ratio at two to one for males over females. Typically, men between sixty-five and seventy-five and those in their teens and twenties (a recent phenomenon) tend to be at the highest risk.

My resident didn't think Juan was serious about killing himself. I wasn't so sure. That's what happens to your diagnostic confidence when you find out that you saw a patient with thoughts of harming himself who later committed suicide. A few years ago, I treated a twenty-year-old man who had been brought in by two police officers after he tried to jump off the Bloor Viaduct, a bridge in downtown Toronto that was a well-known suicide magnet (a security barrier added since then has made jumping off the bridge impossible).

The young man the police brought in was talked out of jumping by a pedestrian crossing the viaduct. The man's mother, who came in as soon as the police told her what had happened, said her son had tried to kill himself twice before. He had spent some time at a psychiatric facility after both attempts. She had thought a new medication program had neutralized his suicidal thoughts. Now she knew they had resurfaced. She asked me to make sure that the psychiatric hospital where he was going to be sent would not let him go home.

"I can't handle him," she said. "I won't be able to stop him if he . . ." She was crying and obviously drained of hope and energy.

"I agree," one of the police officers said to me. "My gut tells me he'll just try again."

My gut was saying the same thing. "I concur," I said. "But it's not up to me."

After sending the patient to the psychiatric hospital, I telephoned and told them how concrened I was. A few days later I learned they had let him go soon after he arrived, and he had indeed killed himself not long after. He had gone back to the bridge and this time had been successful. The police officer came to see me when he found out. I have known this officer for years and had seen him on many occasions. A man in his mid-fifties who was ordinarily respectful and pleasant, he now spoke quickly and loudly. He paced as he poured out his frustration at the young man's death. His hands were shaking. He couldn't believe the man had been sent home yet again. My hands were shaking too. That doesn't happen often to me.

It didn't have to go that way, but it did. We have sent patients home from Mount Sinai and found out later that things didn't go as we hoped, so I'm not pointing fingers. It happens. You just wish it didn't.

Overall, Juan certainly seemed to fit the pattern of someone at risk to commit suicide—even more so than the twenty-year-old I'd sent to the same psychiatric hospital a few years ago. I asked my resident if she knew the SAD PERSONS Scale, a clunky acronym for a list of ten questions designed to help medical professionals assess whether a patient is potentially suicidal. Since its introduction in 1983, it has proven to be a helpful tool, although it is by no means foolproof. "A group of medical students who were taught SAD PERSONS demonstrated a significantly greater ability to accurately evaluate and make recommendations for disposition of a low-risk and a high-risk patient, as judged by three experienced psychiatrists," it was reported in *Psychosomatics,* the official journal of the Academy of Psychosomatic Medicine.

The resident had heard of SAD PERSONS but had not applied it in Juan's case. "I forgot, I guess," she said.

We went over the ten questions in the scale. Each yes answer is awarded a point; a score of 1 or 2 indicates low risk, 3 to 5 indicates moderate, and 6 to 10 signals high:

Sex (if male, award a point)
Age (if less than 19 or greater than 45 years, award, a point)
Depression (patient admits to depression or decreased
concentration, sleep, appetite and/or libido)
Previous suicide attempt or psychiatric care
Excessive alcohol or drug use
Rational thinking loss, psychosis, organic brain syndrome
Separated, divorced or widowed
Organized plan or serious attempt
No social supports
Sickness, chronic disease

Based on what we knew, Juan scored at least a 6 (Sex, Age, Depression, Excessive drinking, Separated and No social support). We didn't know if he had ever tried to kill himself before or, if so, whether it had been organized/planned, and we weren't sure if he had suffered any rational thinking loss. It didn't seem as if he had a serious sickness but it couldn't be ruled out. "I think he's a risk to do himself in," I said, based as much on what the resident had told me as on the tally from the SAD PERSONS Scale.

When I entered his room Juan was lying on his side facing a wall. He was holding his pillow in his arms, like a child cuddling a doll. I asked him to turn on his other side, but he didn't respond. "I'm going to move your bed then," I said, "so we can talk better." As I went to do this he rolled over and faced me.

"You had a rough night, huh?" He grunted a yes. "This happen before? The binge drinking?" Another grunt. "Do you think you have a problem with alcohol?"

"I was off the booze, cold turkey, for six months before . . ." he said.

"Before your girlfriend left you." He nodded. "You have anyone you can talk to? Someone close to you?" I asked.

"I'm all alone, man," he said, almost tearing up.

"Would you be willing to go over to the psychiatric hospital? They have people there who you can talk to."

"I don't think so," he said after a brief pause that made me think he was mulling it over. "I just want to go home."

"I'm worried about you," I said, choosing my words carefully. "I'm concerned about you. I want to make sure you don't do something foolish, like kill yourself. You ever thought about killing yourself?"

"Maybe."

"You ever tried it before?"

"No. Not unless you count drinking too much." He laughed a little when he said this.

"Actually I do," I said. "You can die from alcohol poisoning. Or step in front of a car because you're too drunk to walk straight.

Or pick a fight with the wrong person. I've seen all that happen to people who were determined to drink themselves into a stupor, like you did tonight."

He was listening to what I had to say. A good sign. Time for a tough, direct question: "Do you want to die?"

A beat, as he thought of his answer. "What do I have to live for?"

Now a beat on my part. He was a fifty-nine-year-old obese man who seemed to have no friends or family. His girlfriend had left him, and his income was precarious. What was the right answer?

"You found a girlfriend to love. You can find another. You were in recovery for six months. You can do it again. But it probably won't happen unless you have help. I don't think you can do it on your own. Do you?"

He shook his head to indicate he agreed.

"I'm a doctor. You came here for help. My best help is to send you over to the psychiatric facility. That's my medical advice to you."

He didn't say yes, but he didn't say no.

"You'll go?"

He slowly nodded a yes.

"Good decision, Juan," I said, and patted him lightly on his shoulder. Although it was an automatic gesture, when I think of it now I know it was an entirely appropriate touch. "I'll get the paperwork ready and we can have a nurse take you over there right away."

I left the room as he began to dress, and asked a security guard to keep an eye on him to make sure he didn't have a change of mind and bolt. We occasionally have patients just get up and leave. The ones who do this before we get a chance to assess them are known as LWBS: "left without being seen." At busy and overcrowded ERs, if wait times are too long, that number can be as high as 10 percent. The other main group is referred to as LAMA: "left against medical advice." These are people we have triaged and begun to treat but who decided they wanted to leave. If patients want to leave, we ask them to sign a form that absolves the hospital from any responsibility for what happens to them after they are out of our care.

As I filled out the paperwork to send Juan to the psychiatric hospital, I spoke to the resident about what had just taken place. She could see that he was far better off being sent to a psychiatrist and that he actually seemed relieved that he wouldn't be going out in the world alone, at least not right away.

"What convinced you that he'd agree to go?" she asked.

It was a good question, another sign that she would be a very good doctor. She wasn't afraid to learn, nor was she fearful of being wrong. That's perhaps the most important quality in a resident, and in any medical profession for that matter. I am always nervous around residents who think they can't make a mistake or show any confusion. The truth is that they will make mistakes; we all do. How they respond to their mistakes is what matters in the long run. Residents who are afraid of being wrong will rarely listen to advice that challenges their decisions, especially from someone they consider a junior, such as a nurse. "When I first started out I thought I would lose face if I admitted I didn't know something," a resident once told me. "I quickly learned the opposite was true. I gained respect with the nurses and doctors when I was truthful about what I knew and didn't know."

I admired her willingness to be reflective and even self-critical. "Go take a couple of minutes and have a coffee or a snack," I said. "You've earned it. We all get tired and at times we all need someone to help us make the best decision possible."

4:52 A.M.

The resident stopped by my office to say the psychiatric hospital had agreed to receive Juan. Meanwhile, the security guard remained seated outside his door. When it came time to transfer Juan, the guard and a nurse accompanied him. We don't do that to embarrass patients, but sometimes they have second thoughts about seeing a psychiatrist. We've had patients who've bolted from the taxi en route to the psychiatric hospital. Bitter experience teaches you to take every precaution.

I asked my resident what, if anything, she had learned from my exchange with Juan. She took a minute to gather her answer. "You seemed to understand him as a person," she said. "I think I just saw him as a patient. You figured him out, whereas I was just asking him questions and not really piecing everything together. I was tired, which I know isn't an excuse, and I think I just didn't put as much energy into it as I could have, probably because he didn't seem to be that sick compared to most of the others here tonight."

The truth is, as I first walked into Juan's room, I saw him as just another unhappy middle-aged man. On another night, that might have been the end of it. But, for reasons I can't completely fathom, his sadness touched me. Perhaps, in my own darkest days, I've felt as lonely as he did at that hour. For whatever reason, in that moment I was able to ignore the whining and hear something else.

What I heard was a cry for help.

CHAPTER ELEVEN

SOMETHING BAD WILL HAPPEN EVERY FEW YEARS

5:00 A.M.

One of the nurses came to my office to ask if I could attend to Jason as quickly as possible. "He's in a lot of pain," she said. "His testicles are grossly swollen." She was a very caring and responsible person, and I trusted that if she wanted me to put him next on the list I should follow her suggestion.

When I entered Jason's room I could see from his posture that the nurse had not been exaggerating. Jason was sitting on the bed, his knees in the air, his legs spread apart. There was a look of absolute anguish on his face.

In his late fifties, Jason was soft around the middle and had pasty skin. He was accompanied by a woman who looked considerably younger than Jason. She left the room when I arrived and stood out in the hallway.

I asked him to show me his scrotum and he had no hesitation doing so. Men are often a little shy about doing this, but he was in such agony that privacy mattered little, if at all. His scrotum was red and had swollen to what looked to be about three times its normal size.

"When did this happen?" I asked him.

Jason explained that it began earlier in the day. "I thought it would go away," he said, "but it didn't."

At this point, I worried that Jason had testicular torsion. It's a condition in which the testicle twists around and around until its circulation is cut off. This is a surgical emergency. A surgeon (usually a urologist) has roughly six hours from the moment the circulation is completely cut off to take the patient to the operating room and untwist it before the testicle dies.

Torsion is a diagnosis in which hours and even minutes count. I pressed Jason to try and remember exactly when the pain had started.

"Maybe ten hours ago," Jason answered. If he did have torsion, this was a long time for it to have been going on.

My instinct, though, told me he didn't have torsion. I placed my money on a condition called epididymitis. The epididymis is a coiled-tube structure located along the back of the testis. It allows for the storage, maturation and transport of sperm. Epididymitis occurs when the epididymis gets infected. Infection can lead to the formation of an abscess, or a collection of pus, inside the scrotum. Epididymitis is nothing to trifle with. I've seen men develop septi-cemia, an infection of the bloodstream, from this condition. But it's not torsion, and so there's no deadline to save the testicle.

The other, less likely possibility was that Jason had Fournier's gangrene, a rapidly progressive bacterial infection of the scrotum and penis. I doubted that possibility, since Jason didn't look sick enough to have that condition.

That I didn't know for sure whether Jason had epididymitis, Fournier's gangrene or torsion placed me in a terrible dilemma. If

I wasted too much time making the diagnosis and calling in a surgeon, Jason might lose his testicle. And I might get sued for negligence. I was tempted to call the urologist to see the patient right away. On the other hand, in my view there's an unwritten rule in the ER that if you haul a specialist out of bed to see a patient in the middle of the night, there had better be a good reason, and epididymitis did not count as one. If the surgeon concludes that your request for an immediate consultation in the middle of the night is inappropriate, he will be reluctant to come quickly the next time you need him.

From time to time, I've spoken to surgeons and surgical residents who refuse to see the patient unless my diagnosis has been confirmed with a CT scan or an ultrasound. This behaviour is so common that many of us in the ER don't even bother making a referral until we've ordered a confirmatory scan.

This is not a problem if the undiagnosed disease progresses slowly enough that you have time to order tests to confirm the diagnosis. It's a different story altogether when you're talking about saving a testicle and time is slipping away. By the time you see the patient, order the ultrasound, wait for it to be done, and wait for a radiologist to give you a report, the window of opportunity to save the testicle may have come and gone. And when the urologist comes to see the patient, if the testicle is dead, he or she will probably chastise you for not calling them sooner!

Unfortunately, I had one such personal experience when I decided to go for an ultrasound instead of calling for a urologist because I thought the risk of torsion was low. Many of my ER colleagues and I have had cases like that. As a result, ER physicians are encouraged to call the urologist before ordering an ultrasound, sleep disruption or not.

There was something else about Jason that caught my attention.

Epididymitis usually occurs in men aged nineteen to forty. Jason was well into his fifties. The big question on my mind was, how the heck did Jason get that infection?

You may not know this, but we check every bit of information patients tell us against our own knowledge and experience. From one moment to the next, we may be making judgments about you and your lifestyle. Epididymitis is a textbook example of judgment on the fly.

If you contract the disease and are under thirty-five and sexually active, we assume, based on experience, that the cause is a sexually transmitted bacterium, either *Chlamydia trachomatis* (chlamydia) or *Neisseria gonorrhoeae* (gonorrhea). Whether we tell you on the spot what we're thinking depends on whether you're alone or with your "monogamous partner."

If, like Jason, you're older than forty, then we assume that the condition is caused by bacteria such as *E. coli* and *Pseudomonas,* which come from an infection of the bladder or the prostate. Sometimes when older men get epididymitis, they may have an underlying cancer of the prostate or the bladder. So, whenever I see an older man with epididymitis, I refer him to a urologist as an outpatient for further testing.

Keep in mind, though, that these so-called rules have all kinds of exceptions. There's nothing to stop a randy middle-aged man from having epididymitis caused by a sexually transmitted disease, just as there's nothing to stop a younger man from having epididymitis caused by *E. coli.*

A highly respected ER colleague misdiagnosed my own case of appendicitis based at least partly on a rule. It was early November 1981, and at the time I was a resident in internal medicine. I had just started a rotation in neurology at Sunnybrook Health Sciences

Centre in Toronto when I developed a mild bellyache. Over a day or so, I limped around with vague discomfort and a bit of nausea. It was so unusual for me to be sick that I just assumed I'd get better without any help.

Two days later, I realized my health wasn't improving, so I checked into Mount Sinai's ER. This was two and a half years before I joined the staff. In fact, it was the first time I'd ever set foot in that ER.

A first-year resident in internal medicine saw me. You could tell what he was training to be by the way he was dressed. He wore a lab coat, but underneath you could see he was wearing a nicely pressed shirt and a sharp tie. Surgery residents always wear greens. Psychiatry residents wear the sharp clothes, minus the lab coat.

The resident was pleasant, thorough and clueless. He poked around my abdomen with the virginal hands of someone who had never diagnosed an acute surgical abdomen in his life. I imagined that, as a resident in internal medicine, he fancied being a cardiologist and looked forward to the day when he could leave belly exams behind forever.

When a young man such as I was way back then comes to the ER complaining of belly pain, if you're not thinking about appendicitis you should look for another job. I'm not being sexist here. Women get appendicitis too, but unlike men they also get ectopic pregnancies and ruptured ovarian cysts, not to mention twisted ovaries. When you see a young woman with belly pain you have all these other potentially serious diagnoses to think of. It's so much easier when your patient is male.

As a wise ER doc once told me, "A young man who comes to the ER with belly pain has appendicitis until proven otherwise." Those are words to practise emergency medicine by. It doesn't mean

that every guy in his twenties and thirties has it, but at least you need
to consider the diagnosis. For women the principle is the same. If
a woman of childbearing potential comes to the ER with belly pain
and you're not thinking "rule out ectopic pregnancy," you're apt to
miss it one day, with disastrous consequences.

These are what we call "patterns of presentation." A young
woman who smokes cigarettes and is on the birth control pill comes
to the ER complaining of chest pain. The ER physician wonders
immediately if she has a pulmonary embolus (PE). That's because
PE is much more common in women who smoke cigarettes and
are on an oral contraceptive that contains estrogen. Quick pattern
recognition is so automatic doctors don't even realize when we're
doing it.

As doctors learn how to diagnose medical conditions, they
memorize collections of symptoms that make up the typical pattern of a disease. In the case of appendicitis, the usual pattern is
for a patient to develop vague discomfort in the upper part of the
abdomen that moves over a few hours to the right lower abdomen.
Appetite decreases, and as the condition progresses, the sufferer
develops nausea and vomiting, and often fever.

Today, if I think a patient has appendicitis, I confirm the diagnosis with a CT scan of the abdomen. Back in 1981, when CT
scans that took pictures of the abdomen were not available, a doctor diagnosed appendicitis not with a fancy X-ray machine but with
her hands and her gut. Turns out, however, that the gut is a lot less
accurate than a CT scan.

When surgeons used to take patients to the operating room
based on their clinical suspicions, in up to 20 percent of operations
they discovered the appendix was normal. In other words, the patient
turned out to have some other condition masquerading as appendicitis. Those included intestinal infections and mesenteric adenitis, a

condition that causes swollen lymph glands in the belly cavity. How important is a CT scan to the diagnosis of appendicitis? Today, the routine ordering of CT scans has reduced the rate of unnecessary appendectomies from 20 percent to less than 5 percent.

When the resident was finished examining me, he brought the staff ER physician to my bedside. Two and a half years later, that person could have been me. That evening it was Dr. Eric Letovsky, later the head of the division of emergency medicine at the University of Toronto and one of the founders of emergency medicine in Canada. He has often been called the "Conscience of the ER." He's one of the smartest, most caring physicians I have ever met.

Letovsky stood beside my stretcher as the young resident recited my history and what he'd found when he examined me. Not much older than the resident, Letovsky examined my abdomen himself. The look on his face told me he was trying to figure out whether I had appendicitis or not.

"Are you hungry?" he asked me.

"Yes," I replied.

"Well, then," he said, "you probably don't have appendicitis."

Letovsky sent me home, advising me to come back if my pain got worse. That evening, a homing instinct made me pine for my mother's cooking. I gobbled down a plateful of roast beef, potatoes and peas and went to bed. By three in the morning my belly pain was much worse, and I started vomiting. That morning, I drove myself to Sunnybrook Health Sciences Centre and checked into their ER. Later that day, a surgeon took out my inflamed appendix.

Letovsky's instinct would be right—in most instances. But some patients with appendicitis *do* have an appetite. That's the thing about medicine: you've got to know when to cling to a rule and when to jettison it.

After I recovered, I called Letovsky to let him know I had had appendicitis after all. He was glad that I was fine. But I wondered if he was bothered that I had let him know his diagnosis was incorrect. Physicians love telling stories about other doctors' booboos, but we're not so quick to relish an anecdote when the joke's on us.

Turns out it was more my discomfort than his. Years later, Letovsky was named the chief of the emergency department at Credit Valley Hospital in Mississauga, Ontario. We gave him a "roast" as a going away gift. I got up and told the story of how the great Eric Letovsky missed my appendicitis.

"Wait a minute," said Linda Jepson, a veteran nurse at Mount Sinai's emergency department. "He missed mine too!" Jepson ran up to the microphone to tell her missed appendicitis story.

Letovsky sat off to the side, laughing until there were tears in his eyes. His ability to laugh at his own human frailty made me love the guy so much more than when I thought that he thought he was perfect.

The fact is, even today, with 24/7 access to CT scans, the brightest, most clinically astute ER physicians and surgeons still misdiagnose appendicitis from time to time.

Here's another thing about the rules. If you don't pay attention to new knowledge in medicine, you might overlook the fact that rules can change over time. A wise mentor once told me how he kept the rules in perspective. "There are only two rules in medicine," he said. "Never say *always* and never say *never.*"

All these thoughts rushed through my head as I thought about Jason. If he had torsion, he needed emergency surgery right away. If he had an abscess, he probably required surgery to drain it, but that could wait until the morning.

I told Jason I thought he had epididymitis, not torsion, and that I would have the nurse give him a narcotic painkiller to help manage his discomfort. He wasn't asking me many questions, which I found unusual. I assumed he was either in too much pain or he just didn't want to know anything more than he had to.

"Is he going to be okay?" the woman with him asked when I left Jason's room.

"I think so," I said. In truth I wasn't certain, but I hate speculating on what I can't see with my own two eyes. In the back of my mind there was a third possibility that I didn't want to miss: testicular cancer. It's relatively rare in a man in his fifties, yet not impossible. All that I knew for certain was that Jason needed to be seen as soon as possible and that I didn't want to make the wrong diagnosis.

———————————

I believe one of our responsibilities is to create a culture of safety in hospitals and doctors' offices. We need to help patients feel they are in a place where not only will they be helped with whatever problem has brought them there, but that they will be listened to by someone who respects what they have to say. I don't think the latter can occur if the doctors dealing with them feel incapable of admitting they might be wrong, or might have erred.

I can't tell you how many times in a gathering of my colleagues I have realized I was the only person talking about having made mistakes. And as I did, I could see a tight little smile on my listeners' faces that signalled to me they were uncomfortable with what I was doing.

Doctors tend to rationalize their mistakes. One way is by referring to them by such euphemisms as "bad outcomes"—similar to the way the U.S. army calls civilian casualties "collateral damage."

One way to protect ourselves from making mistakes is to do what's called the "million-dollar workup." The doctor orders every possible test and procedure for a patient so that if something later goes wrong, he can trumpet that he did everything he could. "Sometimes things happen," he can say, "even when every base has been covered."

For example, a patient comes in with chest pain. The doctor orders three sets of blood tests, well spaced apart, to rule out a heart attack. He conducts a nuclear medicine scan to rule out a blood clot. Next he orders a CT scan to rule out a dissected aorta. By the time the patient leaves the hospital, she is irradiated, toxic and shell-shocked. A huge load of public money has been spent. And all along, what did the symptoms and the doctor's gut and experience tell him was actually wrong with her? She had indigestion.

I know our profession does a lot of things right, and that in general patients receive excellent care and treatment when they enter our hospitals. But not always, which is a reality health professionals need to accept. According to the 2004 Canadian Adverse Events Study, 7.5 percent of hospital admissions are associated with medical errors. With an estimated 2.5 million hospital admissions annually, that means 185,000 hospital admissions each year are associated with an adverse event. According to the same study, between 9,250 and 23,750 deaths due to preventable medical errors occur at Canadian hospitals annually.

In 2007, the Canadian Institute for Health Information (CIHI) released a study of what happens to people when they enter a Canadian hospital. The chance of an adult contracting an infection while in an acute care hospital was about one in ten, while the possibility of a child contracting an infection while in hospital was about one in twelve. That study also found that more than 70 percent of nurses and 80 percent of hospital administrators say patients are likely to have a serious medical error while receiving treatment at a Canadian hospital.

When a passenger jet crashes it makes headlines. When someone dies because of a medical error, in most cases no one but the family, doctors and nurses involved seems to notice. I think we should. Up to sixty-five people die *every day* because of mistakes in Canadian hospitals. Compare that to the average number of people who die in air crashes: fifty-two *every year.*

Medical errors are obviously devastating to patients and their families. Fortunately the vast majority are caught in time or do not harm patients, but some do. When doctors and nurses use dispassionate terms such as *adverse events, sequelae,* or *unfortunate outcomes* to talk about bad things that happen to patients, you might think they don't care, or worse. A classic example is the doctor played by Alec Baldwin in the film *Malice.* Arrogant and inevitably dangerous to his patients, Baldwin's character says in response to a question posed during a malpractice trial: "You ask me if I have a God complex. Let me tell you something. I *am* God."

He was wrong. Doctors are not God, of course, and thankfully I have met few who actually think this way, although some might qualify as God wannabes.

A few doctors have over the years been willing to talk about their mistakes. One is Dr. Ellen Anderson Penno, an ophthalmologist in Calgary, who is willing to discuss the time she failed to diagnose a brain tumour called a meningioma.

"I actually missed [it] for a period of time," she told me on *White Coat, Black Art.* "The patient came in repeatedly. Her vision wasn't quite up to snuff. Things looked 'flat.' I did visual tests, visual fields. I could not find any objective findings other than her complaints. Finally, the family doctor and I talked and he said, 'Let's scan her,' because she kept complaining. She had a large meningioma in her orbit. The outcome was generally good, but that deserved a big apology on my part. Although I couldn't find anything, I wasn't listening carefully enough to the patient's symptoms."

I have found that patients and their families are often willing to forgive you when you admit you've made a mistake. What they won't forgive, however, is your not telling them what you did wrong, or making up an excuse for what happened.

There is an even greater potential for mistakes in the ER than in a hospital proper. That's because the relentless pace and constant time pressure in the ER contribute to the risk of medical error. Just about every ER doctor and nurse I've met has a personal story of a mistake. Any of us can describe that long, lonely walk to the patient's bedside to fess up.

All of us deal with the haunting words "what if." *What if* I'd remembered to do this? *What if* I hadn't done that? In most other lines of work it's relatively easy to move on after a mistake. We can't do that in hospitals and medical clinics.

"Some poor guy came in and he was autistic and about thirty years old," Dr. Bruce Campana of Vancouver General Hospital told me on *White Coat, Black Art*. "He was brought in screaming and violent, and he would try to reach out and grab people. The care woman came and said, 'Look, he always gets like this when he is constipated. Can you just give him an enema and get him out of here?' We gave him an enema. The guy was still screaming and yelling. The care people said, 'This always happens. Can we just take him home?' So he went home. I came in for the next shift. You know that feeling when somebody looks up and they say those fateful words: *Do you remember that patient you saw last night? He's dead.* He, of course, had a ruptured appendix."

I asked Dr. Jerome Groopman, a Harvard professor and the author of *How Doctors Think,* to analyze the mistakes committed by Dr. Campana and his colleagues when they looked after the man with autism.

"These are some of the hardest patients to take care of: people who are mentally ill, people who have developmental disorders like autism, and so on," Groopman told me on *White Coat, Black Art*. "First, let's start with what is called a *framing error*. So this thirty-year-old autistic man is put in the frame of 'constipation': he's often constipated. We also have an availability error, meaning that what first came to mind is the diagnosis that occurred in the past. He's been constipated in the past. This is the same pattern so it's the same thing. That's what is most available in your mind. That also causes a cascade of what is called *diagnosis momentum*—it's like a boulder rolling down a hill gathering force. This is what it is; this is what it has been in the past. There is also what is called an *attribution error,* and that is on the emotional side. We tend to find difficult patients [such as] people who we can't connect with emotionally, like autistic people or mentally ill people, difficult to handle. We don't like them often when we are physicians because they make our lives much more difficult. It is difficult to get a history from this man. So we are more apt to quickly attribute whatever is going on to this stereotype that we have, which is a flailing autistic man, and we want to get him out of the emergency department as quickly as possible. All of those factors in thinking and feeling coalesced to cause this tragedy."

One of the key ways doctors can counteract the kinds of problems that occurred with the autistic patient, said Groopman, is to know what type of errors they are prone to make. This, of course, requires a willingness to admit that we are capable of making such grievous mistakes, a self-awareness that not all my colleagues possess. It especially requires doctors to recognize when they have become irritated or are rushing about in a frenzied state. "You want to resist diagnosis momentum and you also want to take your own emotional temperature," he said. "So wait a minute, let me ask a few questions of myself and of the family and let me see where that takes me.' That pause can make the difference between life and death."

If you as a patient, or as someone accompanying a patient in the ER, sense the doctor or nurse is jumping to conclusions or not taking all the factors you believe are relevant into consideration, you have a right to intervene. You have a right to say, "It seems to me you're rushing this a bit. Can we just slow down a second here?" Every medical professional will react to this in their own way—some, frankly, will not welcome your intrusion—but many will listen and perhaps realize that you've offered some valuable feedback. I know that any time a patient or their loved one challenges me I listen. It can get my back up at times, but I also know I am capable of becoming speedy during a long shift. A word or two from a patient can be enough to slow me down a moment. Even if I decide what she says is bunk, I need to stop and gather my thoughts to explain why it's bunk. And in doing so perhaps I might occasionally realize she's right.

The CIHI study found something else: your chance of being given the wrong medication in a hospital is about one in ten. That doesn't surprise Dr. Beverley Orser, an anaesthesiologist and one of Canada's foremost experts in cataloguing problems that lead to medication errors. She was part of a survey that asked members of the Canadian Anaesthetists' Society whether they had been involved in any such errors.

"We were surprised by the answers we got back," she told me on *White Coat, Black Art*. "The vast majority, 85 percent, had been involved with either medication error or a near miss. Now, most were inconsequential and not associated with any morbidity or problems. But there were a number of serious medication errors and

four deaths reported. I don't know over what time period. Anaesthetists know [what they administer] are potent drugs and they need
to be very cautious about it. We think we have to put this in context.
Given the number of medications that are delivered during the day,
and we estimate there are over 40 million patients anaesthetized in
North America alone each year, the incidence is quite low. We can't
overstate that anaesthesia is safe, the systems are safe, but there is
certainly room for improvement."

If you have surgery scheduled please don't cancel it. I am not
saying that what doctors and nurses do is unsafe. However, I don't
think it's as safe as it could be. My theory about why doctors are
so uncomfortable talking about medical mistakes is that they don't
know how to deal with them in a healthy way and can be brutal to
colleagues who make mistakes.

"Every doctor lives in mortal fear of making a mistake," says Dr.
Jerome Groopman. "But being [yelled at and being] afraid of making mistakes doesn't teach you how not to make mistakes. Mistakes
need to be understood, and you need to give people a vocabulary in
terms of what kinds of mistakes occur and a strategy to improve your
diagnostic and treatment skills."

Dr. Bruce Campana was involved in a different kind of yelling
in 2006 when he led a public outcry against his own ER department
at Vancouver General Hospital (VGH), a protest that was echoed
by doctors in two other Vancouver hospitals, Lions Gate and Royal
Columbian.

Campana and a majority of the other ER doctors at VGH
signed an open letter to the public expressing non-confidence in
their ER and provided examples of the types of things that happen
to "real patients from a typical shift." The letter noted that a chest
pain patient who was later found to have suffered a heart attack had
been left in the ER hallway for hours. That a bowel cancer patient

writhed in pain for two hours because he couldn't be given morphine in a hallway. And that an elderly woman was left in her own excrement for a lengthy period in the hallway.

"Let me be clear on this," Campana wrote in a letter to a local newspaper. "People are suffering and dying in the emergency departments because of overcrowding and an insufficient number of doctors and nurses. Our continuous quality improvement director reported one such death last week."

That death, *CTV News* reported, involved a woman who waited three hours in the ER hallway before getting a bed. The bed was secured following a blood test showing she'd had a heart attack. The woman died less than two hours later. Optimally, says Campana, she'd have been put in a monitored bed immediately upon her arrival in hospital. Campana makes it clear he blames the situation on inadequate funding, not failures by staff at VGH.

Following such a drastic move—everyone who signed the letter was risking his or her career—the B.C. government downplayed its concerns and blamed any problems on previous governments.

I'm comforted in knowing that the problems Campana and his colleagues outlined are not typical of Mount Sinai, although we are far from perfect. Fact is, sooner or later, every hospital will have incidents like the one he wrote about.

Hate to say it, but many of us experience *schadenfreude* when talking about colleagues' medical mistakes. No one admits it, so I will now. Sometimes, it's delicious to hear about another ER doc's mistake. In fact, dissing the other guy's medical care is a tradition in medicine. Heck, Hollywood producers named a popular TV show in the 1980s with that concept in mind. The show was called *St. Elsewhere,* and it was about the lives and work of the staff of the fictional St. Eligius Hospital, a rundown, unreputed teaching hospital in Boston. The show starred famed American actor and future double

Academy Award-winner Denzel Washington, not to mention Canadian comic Howie Mandel, a kid I knew growing up in Toronto.

"St. Elsewhere" is a term used by doctors to talk about a hospital other than the one they work at, where malpractice occurs on a regular basis. In the pilot episode of the series, Dr. Mark Craig, played by William Daniels, tells colleagues that St. Eligius has been dubbed "St. Elsewhere" because it's "a dumping ground, a place you wouldn't want to send your mother-in-law."

At Mount Sinai we tend to refer to other hospitals as "Elsewhere General." But you get the idea. When doctors present a patient they've saved, it adds a bit of fun and spice to the presentation if they can say that the patient was misdiagnosed at "Elsewhere General" before coming to their hospital.

I've always hated the arrogance that goes into saying—and, worse, believing—that the other doctor always makes mistakes but that I never do. It's wrong. If you practise real medicine in the real world, you make mistakes. You forget to ask a question. You order an antibiotic without checking to see if the patient is allergic to it.

More than that, what I hate especially are the ER colleagues who pretend they only made mistakes during their first few years of practice, that somehow they became so wise and so experienced they never made another mistake again. Sure, experience helps. But it's not bulletproof. Dr. Romeo Bruni, a wise ER colleague, once told me that "something bad will happen every three or four years." And you know what? He's right. Once or twice every few years, I have a "bad outcome" that will haunt me for the rest of my life. And no, they didn't all happen twenty years ago.

One time I saw a young man who came in with chest pain and shortness of breath. When I came on duty, I found the ER to be packed with patients.

When paramedics had brought my patient in during the early

afternoon, the triage nurses had noted a faint smell of alcohol on his breath. His heart rate was fast, but they attributed it to the booze.

When I arrived for duty, the nurses were happy to see me. As a veteran ER doc, I know how to move patients quickly through the system and clean the place out. I grabbed my patient's chart. By the time I saw him, he looked a lot more comfortable than the initial description suggested. His heart rate was no longer fast. He did not complain of chest pain or shortness of breath. His troponin, a blood test that detects the first dead heart muscle cells that indicate a myocardial infarction (heart attack) was negative.

I sent the patient home. Two weeks later, he died suddenly in his sleep. The autopsy showed he had cardiomyopathy, a condition that damages and weakens the heart, and that is not considered easily treatable. Medication could have stabilized his condition but would not have eliminated it. The only cure for him would have been a heart transplant, a near impossibility in the short term.

Did he have cardiomyopathy when I saw him? It's a difficult diagnosis to make and is one not often suspected in young, apparently healthy people. His breathing wasn't laboured, and he wasn't sweating. When I listened to his chest, I didn't detect the crackly sound of blood backing up into his lungs. A chest x-ray may or may not have detected an enlarged and failing heart. In that case, I would have referred him to a cardiologist for admission and a full assessment. And he might be alive today.

Later, the case was discussed at our own version of "Morbidity and Mortality" rounds. I know I could have ordered lots more tests. I could have ordered a CT scan looking for a pulmonary embolus or a dissecting aorta. I could have held my patient in the ER until we did several troponin tests to rule out a heart attack definitively. I probably should have ordered a chest X-ray, looking for an enlarged heart and signs of heart failure.

If I had to do it over again, I may have acted differently. I also know that when I arrived that fateful evening, the department was packed, and I was determined to do my bit to get the place moving again. And that was on my mind when I sent my patient home.

That's an example of the private hell I put myself through with every error.

Dr. David Lendrum, an ER physician at a hospital in western Canada, recalls an uncommon incident that occurred as he was starting out in his career: a veteran nurse intervened to protect a patient from an ER doctor she considered incapable of dealing with his patient.

"Emergency docs are kind of voyeurs," he says, "so when a sick patient comes in, a lot of the time we all go to the trauma bay and kind of poke our heads in to see what's going on and, I think for the most part, to make sure that if help is needed we can lend a hand. We're a pretty collegial group."

The incident in question took place about one in the morning and involved a forty something male who had been badly injured in a motorcycle accident. "The medics had tried to put a breathing tube down his throat in the field, tried to intubate him, and they were unsuccessful, so this guy was lying there on the trauma bay table, not doing very well," as Lendrum recalls. "One of the nurses had already come to me and this other staff member and said, 'You know, we don't think [the doctor in charge] is going to do a good job. We're really worried about this patient.'"

It was wintertime, and for some reason—perhaps the patient had been drinking—he had ridden his motorbike in a snowstorm. "I don't know what he hit or what happened, but I know his face was smashed and his chest was smashed, he had low blood pressure, a high heart rate, and he was very, very sick," as Lendrum recounts it.

The man was in serious condition—a CTAS level 1 trauma— and about twenty people had gathered in the trauma bay. Although

Lendrum was a recent graduate he could tell the nurse's instinct had been accurate. The doctor in charge was definitely struggling.

"[He] was clearly uncomfortable and overwhelmed with the situation, in the sense that I don't know if perhaps the severity of the situation wasn't appreciated by him or this patient was so sick he didn't know what needed to be done," according to Lendrum. "And he ordered a drug that would have killed him. There's no two ways about it."

"We had to come to the bedside and go, 'Whoa, whoa, whoa. Hold on,'" Lendrum says. "That was really hard. I had been working there for just five months, so I was very thankful to have one of the senior docs with me to approach the bedside. We were whispering around the nurses, saying, 'Don't you dare give him that drug. Here are the drugs we actually need.' And we totally took over and had to push this doctor out of the way."

The overwhelmed doctor stood aside and allowed his senior colleague and Lendrum to take over. It was, he says, like a football player on the sidelines running onto the field without being asked and replacing the quarterback because the play he was about to call would lose his team the game. Except in this case a bad call probably would have killed the patient. "I was stunned at how dangerous this was," he says. "It wasn't a medicine issue at all. The medicine isn't the challenging part. It's all these administrative and personal issues that come up."

Lendrum and his colleague worked feverishly to stabilize and treat the patient. Within fifteen minutes, they had intubated him, put in a central line and inserted a chest tube. "Looking back on what we did afterwards, it was really something tough, but we got it all done, and I was very proud of that aspect of care. Prior to that, anyone who had reviewed that case would have been like, 'That is malpractice. Catastrophic error.'"

The motorcycle patient had kept Lendrum long past the time when he was supposed to end his shift (he was scheduled to book off just as the case came in). About five minutes after cleaning up, however, the same nurse who had sounded the alarm on the overwhelmed doctor again came up to Lendrum and his senior colleague and told them five people with gunshot wounds had just been brought in. Because of what had just happened, the two of them had to override the attending ER physician again—"No one would even let him into the trauma bay," Lendrum says—and their colleague had to stand by once more as they managed the five wounded patients.

In a situation such as this, which thank God I have never experienced—it's no fun watching a colleague appear to mess up to that degree—the nurses are often the ones who file a report. That's because it's the nurses, not our ER colleagues, who work right alongside us and are thus in a better position to see when we mess up. But it doesn't always happen this way. It's as if there's an unwritten code at some hospitals that only doctors can report on doctors and only nurses can report on nurses.

Though I feel for the colleague who screwed up, I know the courageous and conscientious nurse did the right thing. Unfortunately, I know of some instances in which nurses don't.

If nurses know a medication is wrong or that a patient needs something right away and don't speak up or tell me, out of fear that they don't have the right to interrupt me (they do), that sets my blood boiling. I have an entire ward to deal with when I'm on duty, and I simply can't see or remember everything. Most nurses realize this and try to help me manage this considerable responsibility. But not all.

When I order tests, I need a nurse to let me know when the results come in, or how the patient is responding to my treatment. Some nurses do, but others don't. There are times when I have sixteen, seventeen or even eighteen patients on the go and I can't keep everyone in mind. Every once in a while a nurse or a resident shows me a chart, and I realize I've forgotten the patient was mine. Likewise, if I haven't made a decision on a treatment for a patient after a certain amount of time has passed, I need a nurse to hector me, politely, to do so. I simply might have forgotten that it was on my to-do list. Life on the night shift can be that stressful, which makes a helpful nurse such a gift to work with.

Most nurses take their responsibilities seriously. But some nurses, perhaps those who suffer from burnout, work to rule. They seem to have an attitude that if it's not their official responsibility they don't have to bother with it. If that happens I seethe quietly. Believe me, there can be little point in confronting a nurse in anger. If I tell a nurse off in that way, word can get around the department far faster than a Twitter tweet, and I can be shunned for months. Same goes for nurses criticizing doctors.

I know that I am far from perfect. I will admit when I'm wrong. There are more than a few nurses who have seen me fumble a central line who have probably questioned my competence. But we all have to continue to work with each other and carry on. That fact earns me the right to expect others to act like human beings first and to worry about the official rules and procedures second.

Dr. Bruce Campana, who gets along well with nurses (he married one), thinks another factor that can cause a disconnect between doctors and nurses is the condescending attitude some doctors have toward those who are not MDs. "You will see some doctors who clearly have 'penis-size' problems that interfere with their function at work," he says. "There are some doctors who need to be treated the way doctors were treated fifty years ago [as if they were omnipotent and all-knowing]. I think that is stupid. I can't take care of patients all by myself. I will wade into any situation with a good

nurse beside me. They are better at IVs, working the monitors, getting the medication than I am. The paramedics are better in the field
than I am. They need me to do what I do."

When he does clash with a nurse it is usually a personality issue,
he says, with fear being the underlying cause. "Fear is the most per-
vasive emotion in our society. Usually if somebody is resisting or
giving you a hard time, they are afraid you don't respect them or
you're going to take something from them. I usually have conflict
with nurses because they are disrespectful, sloughing off, not doing
their job. I dislike work aversion. I work pretty hard."

Like me, Campana finds laziness to be a major reason he might
clash with a nurse: "A night is longer when someone isn't doing their
job," he says. He tells of an experienced nurse who was agreeable
to deal with one-on-one but painful to work with. "I had a patient
with renal colic, a kidney stone, which is *very* uncomfortable. I said,
'We need to get Gravol and morphine on IV.' The nurse said okay
and went on her break. She didn't pass this on to another nurse.
She left this guy for fifteen minutes writhing in pain and vomiting. I
had trouble with that. That's the kind of thing she does. She shrugs.
She's far enough gone in burnout and doesn't care. She wants to do
the job and take home the pay and to have her world disturbed as
little as possible. Somebody like that needs to stop working, and she
hasn't realized that."

The nurse in question was the type of person who, if confronted,
would deny having done anything wrong and would aggressively
counterattack. So Campana saw no benefit in challenging her directly.

You might think that a doctor should be able to get rid of a
nurse who acts that callously. But it's not so easy.

He says it's even more difficult for doctors, especially those
working in the U.S., to get rid of a doctor they don't respect. "I
have a buddy who works at a hospital in California who is chief of

staff and [he says] there have been complaints of a surgeon who has killed a number of people," says Campana. "There have been hearings and [yet] he can't get kicked out. Unless a surgeon is butchering people you can't get them out."

In the ever-changing power dynamics that govern an ER (and every workplace has its own dynamics), I think what ultimately determines how well a shift works or, on a broader basis, how well the entire department works, comes down to the competence and the quality of the people who work there. But I believe that it's also the personalities of the people who work in the ER can help make the difference between a positive and a negative environment or a successful and an unsuccessful workplace.

What are the qualities I like most in nurses? I love working with nurses who keep close watch on their patients. They have an intuitive grasp of how sick their patients are, which is more important than book knowledge. They don't report to me each time a patient hiccups. Experience tells me that when they're worried about a patient, it's for a very good reason.

They also act as a filter between the patient and me. They don't ask me to answer questions from the patient that I can't answer, like how long it will take until he can go home. A good nurse who gets heat from the patient or the patient's family doesn't automatically transmit that heat to me.

Another appealing characteristic is to project an air of calm. There's a look of serenity on the nurse's face that says, "I like this job and I like patients." Experience helps nurses acquire that look. And yet some of the best ones have it fresh out of school. It usually takes me about an hour or two to know whether a nurse has serenity or not.

Obviously resources play a big part in how well an ER functions. Clever minds, of which there are many in hospitals, can always find ways to best manage and utilize them. But a lazy, arrogant, cynical, burned-out or difficult person can hamper, hinder and otherwise derail even the most efficient workplace. Blame can't be allotted to any one group, be it nurses, residents, doctors or administrators (although the latter have the greatest potential to mess things up, usually because they have a tendency to impose impractical theories onto a system that desperately needs practical ones, as I see it).

One person with a negative personality not only causes problems, he often infects others. One slow or burned-out doctor or charge nurse can turn a well-run ER into a log-jammed nightmare for the staff and the public. One unco-operative consultant can make a great shift go sour really fast.

I have an ER colleague at Mount Sinai who can see five or more patients an hour. He is driven and relentless. When the nurses don't put patients on chairs and stretchers fast enough, he brings them in from the waiting room himself, sometimes in a conga line procession. Not surprisingly, many of the nurses find it difficult to work with him at such a pace. He works so frenetically that many nurses just can't keep up to him. On the other hand, a much slower doctor can take the quietest shift in a month and turn it into a disaster by seeing just one or two patients an hour. If this happens, the nurses mutter silently under their breath until help in the form of a faster doc—often the very same speedster I talked about—arrives to clear the backlog.

Fortunately, there are lots of solutions. One is to hire more health professionals to help with the load. Recently, our ER hired its first nurse practitioner or NP—a registered nurse who has taken a postgraduate degree in advanced nursing. NPs are licensed to work independently of physicians, albeit with a narrower but useful scope of practice. They can order tests and prescribe medications. When a patient's condition falls outside their scope of practice, they can ask MDs like me for help. Recently, we also hired our first physician assistant or PA. Unlike NPs, PAs must work under the direct supervision of a physician.

As for me, all I can control is myself, so I make it my goal, through my work at the ER and as a journalist (and through this book), to spread the message: we have to put our fears and jealousies and other base traits aside if they interfere with the incredibly vital job we've chosen to take on. Patients must come first. Everyone agrees with that in theory (I pray). In practice, though, it's not always the case.

When it comes to talking about medical mistakes, I'd like to dispel a big misconception that they're always the fault of one person, such as a physician, a nurse or a paramedic who should have known or done better. Nonsense. Many studies have shown that one person is seldom to blame for a medical error.

Take, for instance, the moment I described in Chapter Seven when, dead tired, I ordered diltiazem instead of diazepam for my patient. The nurse who heard my order gently corrected me. Because she caught the error, the patient narrowly avoided getting the wrong medication. Unfortunately sometimes my errors are not caught, resulting in what we call a "system failure."

Not too many years ago, I saw a patient who had fallen off a ladder trying to clean some leaves out of the eavestroughs of her house. A colleague had seen her and ordered X-rays of her spine before handing her off to me and going home. Rather than wait for a resident in radiology to read the films, I read them myself. I misread one of the X-rays quite seriously. It wasn't that I failed to see a broken vertebra. That would have been hard to miss. It's that I failed to appreciate that the vertebra was so badly broken that some of the squashed vertebra had pushed backwards toward the woman's spinal cord. I had checked her more than once for evidence of a spinal cord injury, and she had a completely normal neurological examination. On the basis of my physical examination plus my faulty reading of the X-rays, I sent her home with a prescription for pain relievers.

I'm an ER doc, not a radiologist. I don't get paid to read X-rays; the radiologists do. Like at all hospitals, the practice at Mount Sinai is that I mark my preliminary X-ray interpretation. That way, the radiologist who reads the X-ray can see whether I was right or wrong. If I've missed something serious, there is a system in place to catch my mistake and advise the ER physician on duty to track the patient down and take corrective action.

But no system is perfectly foolproof. In this case, it took longer than usual for my mistake to be detected and for the patient to be contacted. Good thing this happened, since the woman needed surgery to stabilize her spine and prevent her from suffering a serious neurological injury. Near misses like this one demonstrate that we need to tighten communication between ER physicians and radiologists.

After reading this, you might get the idea that you're in mortal danger every time you're admitted to hospital. That's far from the truth. It's just that you need to know the health-care system isn't some all-seeing, all-knowing computer. It's an aggregation of humans with all of their individual frailties.

Since that incident, plus the one involving my young patient who died of cardiomyopathy, I've made it my mission to do my bit to help create a culture of safety in hospitals. My colleagues and I have to get a lot more comfortable as frail humans practising medicine. We need to debrief in a routine, systematic way following each ER shift, each operation and each tour of duty in the ICU. We need to report to each other all of the bad outcomes, the near misses and the things that went according to plan. That way, everyone can benefit from the lessons each of us learns on our own, but that until now we have been reluctant to share.

5:10 A.M.

I phoned the resident who was on-call to the urology service to see when he would be able to see Jason. He was at St. Michael's Hospital prepping a patient for a kidney transplant. He said he'd arrive as soon as possible. That wasn't promising. A kidney transplant sure sounded more urgent than my patient with a swollen testicle. And yet, if as I strongly suspected, Jason had torsion, time was running out before he risked losing his testicle.

I thought about calling the staff urologist on duty. But because I wasn't convinced Jason had torsion, I didn't want the embarrassment of calling a specilaist unnecessarily.

In my opinion, the relationship between ER doctors and specialists (or consultants, as we call them), such as a surgeon with a particular expertise, is a critical and often tricky part of our work. It takes up our time and requires tact and, quite often, a willingness to bite our tongue because some of them regard calls from the ER as a nuisance and an imposition.

There can be, frankly, a considerable divide between ER doctors and consultants; there's an art (and it can be a very black one) to getting a consultant to accept your call and to act quickly when speed is required. Some of us refer to the process of negotiating as "pimping a consult," and the word *pimping* is aptly chosen. Some ER doctors feel they have to puff up a patient's condition to make it seem as urgent as possible (even if it's just semi-urgent); others use flattery to get a specialist to the ER.

Consultants would probably say ER doctors often call them unnecessarily. "Do you have any idea how many times I've been asked to look at someone who had minor abdominal pain?" a surgeon once said to me. "You guys are so afraid of making a mistake that you dump all these patients on us in the middle of the night when there is no reason to send them our way." A false alarm can be annoying, but I think the number of times this happens is small. The consultants don't remember all the calls that were indeed urgent; they have no idea (nor should they, I suppose) just how many times we don't call them, times when we call a minor stomach ache just that.

There is a word consultants use that drives me nuts: "inappropriate." They categorize certain requests for their assistance as inappropriate consults. To me, this is condescending to the patient and to the referring physician. Granted we can be wrong, but the nature of life in the ER is such that we have to act quickly and decisively. Better the consultants are inconvenienced every now and then than we don't call when a patient's health could be at stake. This is the world we have to navigate shift after shift.

As an ER physician I don't control the beds, nor can I make a surgeon come down any faster. These limitations can foster a sense of helplessness at times when it appears that rules that you can't bend as an ER physician can be bent by colleagues who are higher up the ladder. I will never forget an incident involving one of my internist colleagues on morning rounds. He was talking about a junior resident who had accepted a referral (admitted a patient to the hospital) from the ER the night before. The patient was elderly and, in retrospect, it became clear she had been confused and had a psychiatric rather than a medical problem.

The internist, who was surrounded by a team of residents, approached me (I was on duty at the ER) and began his conversation by calling me by my first name. I have learned over time that when they call you by your first name they usually want something. "Brian," he said, "there's this eighty-two-year-old woman who was referred last night. They thought it was a medical problem. Not an unreasonable thing to do. Now we think this patient has a mental health problem and we are handing the patient back to you."

The internist said this last part with a quiet certainty, his tone and demeanour set to impress those he was teaching. The only problem was that he didn't have the authority to hand the patient back to me. Once the consultation had been accepted, he had four options: admit the patient, refer her to another service, request admission to the hospital's intensive care unit if she was critically ill, or send her home. He could return a patient to the care of the ER physician only if it was clearly in her best interests.

This internist happened to be a nice guy, and I was, at the time, too timid to refuse what I knew was an unwarranted transaction. "Shit runs downhill," he said, in a commiserating tone. It took me almost two decades to learn how to say no in these kinds of situations. In the past I didn't want to be seen as a whiny, passive-aggressive kind of colleague. I wanted to be a good guy. Saying yes to requests like that means sticking your neck out. For some reason, emergency physicians tend to do that. But most of us have learned that if we stick our necks out once too often our heads get lopped off.

I remember a colleague who ended up treating a patient who had been advised by his family doctor to go to the ER and ask to be seen by a consultant in the internal medicine service. But the ER physician, knowing that internal medicine had been inundated by consult requests that evening, decided to do the assessment himself. He was too afraid or too considerate to send yet another person to a department that he knew didn't want any more patients at the time. My colleague took the patient's history, conducted a physical examination, assessed that all was well and sent the patient home. Sadly, the patient died soon after; he should have been sent to internal medicine after all. I've often wondered why my colleague didn't do this. Perhaps he felt he had referred too many patients that day and didn't want to abuse the privilege. Perhaps he had low self-esteem and feared being criticized by the consultant.

I know an ER doc in another province who saw a patient with osteomyelitis, an infection of the bone. The condition required surgery and IV antibiotics. Trouble was, though he found an orthopedist willing to do the surgery, he couldn't find an internist willing to put the patient on antibiotics. My colleague got so fed up with having his patient in admission limbo that he arranged to treat her himself in the ER, as an outpatient. He started her on an antibiotic called gentamicin. Unfortunately, she developed two devastating side effects. Two weeks after starting the antibiotic, she began to suffer from oscillopsia, a form of dizziness that became permanent. Worse still, she developed kidney failure, which is also a known side effect of gentamicin. In retrospect, my ER colleague was mad at himself for taking on the responsibility of treating the patient. He felt he got burned for trying to help out a patient who needed a specialist. The saying "No good deed goes unpunished" comes to mind.

I'm happy to say, however, that most of my attempts to get a consultant to respond to my call for help have been positive and satisfactory—but not all. One in particular was so upsetting it was described in a 2008 article entitled "Holiday in Hell" by the *Medical Post*. It was published around Christmas and told of an incident I'd experienced during the holidays a few years earlier.

A man had turned up at Mount Sinai at 1:00 a.m. on Christmas Eve suffering from several complex finger lacerations right down to the tendons, the result of an engine hood mishap. "I couldn't find a plastic surgeon because our plastic surgeon had signed out for Christmas and there was supposed to be an arrangement with another hospital . . . and (that) plastic surgeon wasn't taking any calls," I told the writer. "I spoke to the resident and the resident yelled at me, 'Under no circumstances are you supposed to talk to me!' And then I spoke to the staff fellow. All of them told me I was supposed to be speaking to somebody else. I stopped seeing patients at 7:30 a.m. and it wasn't until noon that I finally got a live human being to say, 'I'll take this patient.'"

The article elicited an angry response from a senior doctor at the hospital I had called for a consult. Without getting into the nitty gritty of his response, let's just say he thought the whole problem was largely my fault for failing to understand all the rules and all the exceptions for which physicians in my ER are permitted to refer to specialists in his department. At times like these, it feels as if the patient is beside the point.

There are situations in which consultants want proof of illness before they agree to see a patient. Then again, in my opinion, there are situations in which they're looking for an excuse to dodge the referral altogether. In a teaching hospital like Mount Sinai, we see that behaviour from time to time in residents who work for consultants.

Most of the time, residents on the consulting services are pleasant, respectful and helpful to ER physicians. However, a few years ago, I was working a night shift when I saw an elderly man with a cough and fever. I suspected he had pneumonia, and I ordered a chest X-ray that confirmed the diagnosis. I felt he needed to be admitted to hospital, and so I requested a consultation with the resident on-call for internal medicine. I called the hospital's switchboard and asked for the resident to be paged. A few moments later, he showed up in the ER. He was tall and thin, and spoke with a fussy kind of voice. I was presenting the history and physical findings of my patient when he suddenly stopped me.

"I'm confused," said the resident. "Why are you calling me to see a patient now?"

I looked at my watch. It was 2:30 a.m. This resident and his team were scheduled to be on-call until 8:00 a.m.

"I'm the one who's confused," I countered. "I'm calling you because I want you to admit my patient."

"Oh, but it's my understanding that we're not supposed to be called with new referrals past 2:00 a.m. unless it's urgent."

"That's not my understanding," I countered.

"Well, if you feel you can't manage your patient, I'll be happy to help. However, only you and one other physician have a reputation for asking for referrals so late," he said. "Most of your colleagues don't seem to need to ask for our services at this time of night."

I smiled as I began to recognize the kind of manipulative skills that parents often see in their teenage children. I decided to respond in kind.

"Well, it's true that I'm getting a little older, and my head's not as sharp as it used to be," I said, maintaining as earnest an expression as I could muster. "I'll be very happy to have your help looking after this patient."

The resident frowned. He had been too clever by half. He was trying to dodge the referral and get me to hold the patient until the next team came on at 8:00 a.m. But his insincere offer of help came back to bite him. He saw the patient. Fortunately for me, his rotation in internal medicine ended soon after. I would have hated having to refer another patient to him.

Invariably there are clashes between physician and residents. My worst encounter with a resident occurred early in my career at

Mount Sinai. I saw a patient one morning who needed to be admitted to the internal medicine service. I paged the resident on call, a smart young woman who had done a rotation in the ER the year before and had now returned as a resident in internal medicine.

When she answered my call, she seemed irritated that I'd bothered her. I began describing the patient's symptoms when she interrupted me with questions that made it difficult to tell her what was wrong with the patient. My antennae went up.

Often, when residents begin asking a lot of questions before hearing the full story, it's because they're listening for answers that will allow them to dodge the consult. The object of the game is for the resident to induce the ER doc to take back the consult. That's because it's a well-recognized ethical principle that attending physicians and their residents cannot refuse to see a patient. In fact, one sure way to get a reluctant resident to see a patient is to threaten to write down on the chart that the resident refused to see the patient.

After a few more questions, I was fairly certain she was trying to dodge the consult. I told her to come down and see the patient. She arrived in the ER hell-bent for conflict. "We are a consulting service," she said, adopting the royal *we* as if she were a charter member. "We aren't here to manage *your* patients. We give *you* advice, and it's up to *you* to manage them."

I was feeling tired and cranky, and the ER was busy. I also had to move on and see to all the other patients I was looking after. "Consult!" I pointed to the room where my patient was and started to walk away.

"Fuck off," she said, within earshot of several patients and staff.

A day or two later, I walked into the ornate office of the chief of internal medicine. I had complained about the resident's attitude and demeanour to the appropriate channels. The chief was a man I respected from medical school days as a smart and ethical physician.

"Before we begin, I should tell you that we think very highly of [the resident]," he said.

The colour drained from my face. I knew where this was going. Her chief was going to back her up on everything, from her attitude to her use of profanity in the course of patient care. And he did. Since this episode, she's become a highly respected consultant in the community. In time, she and I developed a *modus vivendi,* shall we say. I'd like to think the chief reamed her out for using profanity, but that's one conversation I'll probably never know about.

5:18 A.M.

The urology resident remembered to call me back following the kidney transplant at St. Michael's Hospital. He made a faint-hearted effort to get me to hold Jason until the next resident took over at 9:00 a.m. I reminded him of our deal, however, and he agreed to see Jason, albeit reluctantly. He was tired, and I didn't want to abuse him. Still, why should my patient suffer for the resident's fatigue?

As the shift entered what the nurses call the witching hour, I resisted the urge to pop another modafinil to keep me alert. I do worry that one day I'll need three pills, then four, then five. . . .

Everyone who works nights in the ER and elsewhere in the hospital knows what the witching hour is all about. It's the time when the urge to sleep is the greatest. As long as things are hopping, you tend to stay awake. But if there's a lull, the urge to nod off can be irresistible.

I don't know if nurses talk about things like this among themselves. There's only one physician on duty overnight at Mount Sinai and most other ERs, so the only way I'd talk about it with the doctors is to talk to myself. But I know that all of us just want to get through the last couple of hours without having to be at the top of our game. You find yourself hoping that EMS doesn't call in with a CTAS 2 (a patient in danger of imminent cardiac or respiratory arrest). Thing is, no one says it out loud. Call it superstition. But there's a widespread belief, especially among nurses, that as soon as you say, "I hope we don't get a CTAS 2," moments later paramedics will bring in not one but two.

Another thing: night or day, if you happen to notice that the waiting room is empty and the working pace is light, never utter the "Q-word"—as in *quiet*. I've met many a nurse who believes fervently that as soon as you say aloud how quiet the ER is, things will become busier instantly.

———

A street fight had brought my next patient to the ER. He was a man in his early thirties, tall and broad-shouldered, and he spoke with an accent. He explained that after a night of drinking with friends he had left a bar when a fight broke out on the street between a small man and a much larger opponent. "I was army and know how to handle myself," he said, "so I step in to break it up." As he did this, the smaller man, whom my patient had thought he was protecting, punched him in the mouth. "I black out and so I come here, to make sure I am okay," he said.

I guess the little guy didn't like good Samaritans. "How long were you out?" I asked.

"I don't know. A few seconds, maybe."

I had the results of his CT scan, which showed no internal bleeding or any other apparent damage. Apart from a bruise on his face where the punch had landed, he seemed fine. When I relayed this information he didn't seem to care.

"My teeth," he said. "Look at my teeth. I paid 4,400 bucks for those fucking teeth. They better not be hurt."

I asked him to open his mouth, pointing out that I was not a dentist. His teeth looked fine. Quite impressive, actually.

"That's why I come," he said. "It hurts in mouth and if that bastard did anything to my teeth . . ."

He had been waiting for several hours to be assured his teeth were not damaged. That's the only reason he came in. I said they looked normal but advised him to check with his dentist if he had any concerns. I offered him some painkillers but he refused them. I guess if I had spent that much on my teeth I wouldn't wait to see my dentist if I had any worries that something might have happened to them.

As we inched toward the end of the shift, all of us who would be clocking out in the next few hours hoped no major case would come in just before we were due to leave. Not that we wouldn't give it our full attention if one did show up. It's just that as our energy starts to ebb, which it inevitably does in the early morning hours, we prefer to tidy up remaining cases before handing them over to the new crew.

In September 2008, Dr. Steven Friedman, a colleague who worked across the street in the ER at University Health Network, was getting ready to wrap up his shift when paramedics showed up with an overweight man who was in full cardiac arrest. The patient, probably in his mid-sixties, was visiting Toronto with his wife. Some time after five in the morning he had sat up in his hotel bed and told his wife he was experiencing a sudden pain and thought he was going to die. Then he collapsed.

When the paramedics reached his room they found him in ventricular fibrillation, a form of cardiac arrest. The paramedics shocked his heart with a defibrillator and applied CPR for the next thirty minutes, but the man had no pulse.

Friedman says he gave himself a moment to despair at his bad luck, but soon realized he had no choice but to try and save the man. The despair quickly gave way to a rush of adrenaline. "Emerg docs like resuscitation," he says. "The fact is it's exciting to do, and you're trained to do it. And it's what we like to do. But in contrast to [what happens on] TV, most cardiac arrest resuscitations don't end well. Immediately this event perks you up, and what little bit of adrenaline you had in your adrenals gets squirted out up there along with whatever coffee you've just ingested. So you run the resuscitation, and we ran it for an insanely long time, because he'd already been down for thirty minutes with resuscitation in progress, and we ran it for another thirty minutes and went through all the protocols." The resuscitation team administered every type of drug they thought might revive the man, but to no avail. That left the task of telling his wife, a middle-aged woman on holiday away from home, that her husband was dead.

"It's particularly hard to do at any time," Friedman says, "but you're now in this incredibly emotional situation and your body's been put through this marathon of being up for hours and sleepless, and then you've done the sprint of a prolonged resuscitation. It's like a sort of decathlon."

5:24 A.M.

"Dr. Goldman, go to Resus 1 stat."

I tore off to Resus 1, wondering what awaited me. Sophia, my first patient—the seventy-two-year-old woman with metastatic lung cancer whom I'd treated for her first seizure—was being wheeled back into the resuscitation room. She looked as if she was coming out of another seizure. As I tried to size up the situation quickly, I was frankly puzzled.

"Sorry to bother you, Brian," said one of the nurses who was pushing Sophia's stretcher as I ran in. "She was fine, and then this happened."

"Where's the medical resident?" I asked the nurse as I tried to get my bearings.

"They're at a cardiac arrest on the fourteenth floor," she replied. "I didn't think this could wait."

As I looked at Sophia, I knew immediately the nurse was right. My momentary hesitation was understandable. Once we hand over patients, it's hard to get back into the mindset of being on the hook again. Truth is, I'd been up all night, and I was hoping my shift would end quietly. Still, with Sophia's resident doctors occupied trying to save someone else, I knew I had no choice but to pitch in.

As I approached Sophia, she had the same glassy look on her face that I had seen earlier. But this time, there was something very different about her demeanour.

"Sophia," I called out to her. She didn't answer.

I glanced at her vital signs on the heart monitor. I looked at her respiration. She was breathing at forty breaths a minute. You and I breathe fourteen to sixteen times a minute. Forty breaths was an incredibly fast rate, a sign of extreme respiratory distress.

When I listened to Sophia's chest, I could hear breath sounds on the right and none on the left.

As I was formulating my thoughts, Sophia's condition began to deteriorate sharply. Her blood pressure, a solid 120 over 70 five minutes earlier, was now 90 over 40. Her heart rate had climbed to 115 beats per minute, an indication her body was under great stress.

Four nurses—two from the resuscitation room and two from the area where Sophia had been resting comfortably—were busy putting in IVs and taking blood work. I didn't have to tell them to do that; they were well trained. But I felt they were looking at me to do something to bring Sophia back from the jaws of death.

I've been working long enough to know what they expected. When a patient is suffering from acute respiratory distress, at some point you have to consider putting her on a ventilator. That means intubating the patient. But Sophia had metastatic cancer. Her seizure was caused by the lung cancer travelling to her brain. I didn't think it was right to put her on a ventilator when her life expectancy could be measured in months, perhaps even weeks.

"What's her code status?" I asked, hoping she was a Do Not Resuscitate.

"She's full code," answered one of the nurses, meaning that we were to do anything possible to keep her alive.

"I don't think it's right that this woman should wake up on a ventilator in the ICU," I said quietly.

No one said anything. I'm quite certain most nurses would have agreed with me. Did we really want to intubate someone without thinking about it? Did we really want to pull out all the stops for someone who almost assuredly was going to die within a month or so? Still, that's an academic argument. No one likes to have a patient die on his or her watch. Even fewer like to sit by and refuse to do something when they have the power to save a patient, albeit briefly.

Then I remembered Sophia's chest X-ray, the one that showed at least two litres of watery cancerous fluid on the left side of her chest. I wondered if the fluid had caused her condition to deteriorate.

"Did the resident take off the fluid?" I asked one of the nurses who had been assigned to care for Sophia.

"They said they'd do it in the morning," the nurse replied.

Suddenly, everything that had caused Sophia's health to deteriorate so quickly began to make sense. She had accumulated a life-threatening amount of watery fluid on the left side of her chest. Her left lung was so compressed by the fluid it had completely collapsed. The pressure exerted by the fluid had become so great it was pushing Sophia's heart toward the good lung on the right side. I had a desperate idea that might just save Sophia's life—without having to put her on a ventilator.

"Get me a 14-gauge Angiocath, some sterile tubing, a syringe and some local anaesthetic," I barked.

The nurses positioned Sophia onto her right side. Quickly, I disinfected Sophia's back and put some local anaesthetic into the skin of the upper back, right where the fluid was. I mounted a syringe on the Angiocath, and slowly stabbed Sophia's back with the catheter, aspirating on the syringe as I advanced the catheter. Four centimetres into Sophia's chest, cancerous fluid began appearing in the syringe. The catheter was in the right place.

I unscrewed the syringe and connected one end of the sterile tubing to the hub of the catheter, and the other to a one-litre vacuum bottle. As soon as I plunged the needle end of the tubing into the vacuum bottle, a litre of fluid flowed out of Sophia's chest and into the bottle.

Back from the cardiac arrest, Sophia's team of residents had raced to join me in the resuscitation room. They saw the fluid quickly filling the first vacuum bottle. I quickly brought the team up to speed.

"Thanks for holding the fort until we got back," the second-year resident said, catching her breath. She looked at Sophia's vital signs and didn't like what she saw. "She didn't look like this the last time we saw her," she said.

"I gather that," I said to her. "But you know what? She looks better than she did before I started draining the fluid." Sophia did look better. Her respiratory rate had dropped ever so slightly from forty to thirty-five breaths per minute. She looked a bit more comfortable. She was even a bit more alert.

"I think the fluid in Sophia's chest was under so much pressure it was pushing the heart toward the good side of her lungs," I said to the resident.

The resident and I looked at each other, trying to figure out what to do next to help Sophia. "Let's put in a chest tube!" We both said it at exactly the same time.

A chest tube is a flexible plastic tube that is inserted through the side of the chest into the pleural space, the area between the chest wall and the lung. Most of the time, we insert a chest tube to treat pneumothorax, a condition in which air is trapped in the pleural space, causing the lung to collapse. But a chest tube can also be used to drain fluid out of the chest cavity in a hurry.

The resident stepped forward. At this point, Sophia was more her patient than mine. "I'd like to put in the chest tube, that is, unless you mind," she said.

"Have you put many in?" I asked her.

"I've done a couple, but not for a while. Do you mind supervising me?"

Did I mind? That's what I'm here for, I thought to myself.

"Let's get started," I said.

I made sure she knew what she was doing. The resident cleaned and draped the chest. After freezing the skin with local anaesthetic, she used a scalpel to make an incision in the space between the fifth and sixth ribs. She used scissors to dissect down to the inner lining of the chest wall, called the pleura. Then she used forceps to puncture the pleura and guide the tube into the chest cavity. Once she was satisfied the chest tube was in the right position, a nurse connected the end of the tube protruding outside Sophia's chest to a vacuum device.

Within half an hour, another two litres of cancerous fluid had been sucked out of the chest. I ordered another chest X-ray to see how Sophia was doing. It showed that most of the fluid on the left side of the chest had been evacuated and the left lung had begun to re-expand.

"You did good," I told the resident.

"Thanks for the assist."

Not bad for a middle-aged ER doc who sometimes feels as if his best days are behind him. But it would be a while yet before we knew if Sophia was out of imminent danger.

CHAPTER TWELVE

CHECKING OUT

6:20 A.M.

Trying to save Sophia's life did more than make me feel proud to be an ER physician. It got me fully awake. That was a good thing, because I'd spent forty minutes tending to her. In the meantime, several patients had registered. I try to see most of the patients who register during my shift. I don't like leaving lots of unfinished business for the doctor who takes over in the morning.

My next patient was a young woman in her twenties who had been punched in the face at a bar several hours earlier. Her boyfriend, who had been with her during the assault, had brought her in when her nose began to swell up. X-rays determined it was broken, but not badly. If it had been seriously fractured she might have required surgery, but this was as minor a break as I had seen in a long time.

"What happened?" I asked her.

She explained that she had been drinking at a local pub with her boyfriend and her roommate, another woman she had known for a long time. Her female friend got drunk, and on her way back from the washroom punched her in the face. She said this in a rather matter-of-fact tone.

"Why did she hit you?"

"She has always liked Andy," she said, indicating her boyfriend. "She just got hammered, like six or eight beers or so, and was angry or horny, whatever, and she hit me."

"Did you report it to the police?"

"No," she said, in a tone that suggested I was hopelessly confused. "She's my friend. She didn't mean it. To break my nose."

I asked her if she felt safe living in the same space as someone who couldn't control her anger or jealousy. She dismissed my concerns and said her roommate would feel awful about what had happened once she sobered up. By this point I accepted there was nothing more I could say about my concerns for her safety. I gave her some painkillers, told her to ice the nose and said the swelling should come down in about four or five days.

"That's great," she said. "We have a wedding to go to."

"You and Andy," I said.

She nodded, and said the roommate would be going as well. Great, I thought. A wedding, lots of alcohol and these three—a potent combination. I wished her well and left, shaking my head.

To me, the punch in the bar was a warning sign, a possible precursor to even more violence ahead. I would not have felt safe being under the same roof with someone who had this kind of anger toward me. Who knew what the next altercation might involve? To her, it was nothing really, an understandable reaction fuelled by booze. She saw no danger ahead and found my concern to be rather ridiculous, an overreaction by an old worrywart. Maybe she was right, I decided. Maybe she knew her friend would feel such remorse that the incident would never be repeated. If so, why make a big deal out of it? Involve the police and maybe lawyers and divide loyalties among friends and family. What a lot of fuss. It happened, she wasn't badly hurt, and it was over. I wish I could let go of things that easily.

6:42 A.M.

The body and mind are incredibly interrelated, as far as I'm concerned. Jungian analyst Irene Claremont de Castillejo says, "Emotion always has its roots in the unconscious and manifests itself in the body." I'm no psychoanalyst, so I'm not certain if "always" is accurate. But I can say that in my decades as a doctor I've seen a lot of evidence to illustrate the truth of this observation.

I believed my next patient was an example of emotions governing the body. Jenny was in her mid-thirties and had arrived with her husband several hours earlier complaining about something lodged in her throat. "We were at a Chinese restaurant two days ago, the one with the buffets," she said, "and ever since then I haven't been able to clear my throat. It feels as if something's stuck in there. I'm getting really worried about it."

I examined her throat and could see a slight redness on her uvula, the small U-shaped piece of soft tissue that hangs down from the soft palate in back of the tongue. The name comes from *uva,* the Latin word for "grape."

"Can you swallow?" I asked.

"Yes."

"Eat?"

"Yes, but I don't want to."

My intuition told me there was nothing wrong with her physically. Nor was there any apparent evidence that something was caught in her throat. The slight redness was likely caused by her constant attempts to clear whatever she felt was inside her throat. "Globus hystericus" is the medical term for the sensation of having a lump in the throat when there is nothing there. Globus is what doctors call a conversion disorder. Patients who have a conversion disorder often complain of neurological symptoms such as numbness or paralysis. As with globus, no organic cause can be found. But still, you have to look for yourself.

A few months before, at about the same hour, a nurse who was looking after patients in the ambulatory care area of the ER asked if I'd mind seeing a patient immediately even though she wasn't first in line. My ears pricked; unless the patient is dying, most nurses I know are ideologically opposed to letting patients jump the queue.

"Brian, I thought you wouldn't mind seeing her first because she's here with her husband and her baby, and the baby is tired and cranky."

It was only then that I could hear the baby's cries; until then I had been quite successful at tuning them out. I agreed to see the patient, a twenty-eight-year-old woman with a cute but fussy eighteen-month-old toddler squirming in her lap.

"I'm glad you came," the woman said. "I was just about to go home."

"What's going on?" I asked.

"We ate in a restaurant. I ordered bass, and about halfway through I felt something get stuck in my throat. I tried eating bread and drinking water but nothing helped. I went to bed but then I woke up around three. When I realized it wasn't going away, I decided to come here."

"Let's take a look," I said.

Secretly, I was dreading this. To get a good look at the throat, you need to use a tongue depressor to push the tongue well down. Most patients gag and produce so much saliva you can't see anything. Quite often, if a fish bone was present, the patient has managed to dislodge it, but the scratch left by the bone makes it feel as if it's still there. Even if the bone is still present, it's often embedded underneath the lining of the throat, making it next to impossible to see. All too often, the search for a fish bone is a futile forty-minute exercise that ends in me referring the patient to the ear, nose and throat clinic.

This time, though, when I placed a tongue depressor on the woman's tongue, she didn't gag at all. I pressed down firmly and saw a half-inch shard of bone poking out from her left tonsil. Right then and there, I was able to snare it with a pair of forceps.

The woman left the ER cured and happy. I thought about her as I tried to figure out what to do with Jenny. I looked at her chart, which noted she was pregnant and in the early part of her second trimester.

"How's the pregnancy going?"

She told me she'd been sick a lot.

"And really worried," her husband, Steve, added. I thought he was trying to sound concerned, but I detected frustration or some other annoyance in his voice.

I prompted her to talk about her pregnancy, which she seemed eager to do. As she told me about her bouts of sickness she let something revealing slip out. "I don't mind being sick, though," she said. "I'm just so grateful we're pregnant, especially after what happened before."

I took the bait, knowing it had been dangled in front of me. "What happened before?"

Jenny looked away from her husband, her eyes fixed on the floor before she stared straight at me. "I had an abortion."

I made a mental note that "we" were pregnant but "I" had an abortion. I looked back at her and smiled ever so slightly, more of a nod than anything else. From my many years conducting interviews for radio and TV, I knew that if I didn't say anything, just nodded and smiled a little, she would continue to speak. It's a strange characteristic of humans that when presented with silence in a situation where we anticipate a response, most of us keep talking.

Experienced print and broadcast journalists use silence to great effect, especially if someone is not telling the truth or is dealing with a deep emotional issue. Supposedly, they teach this technique in med school, although it's rare to find physicians aside from psychiatrists who actually put it into practice.

Kim Marvel, a family physician and a teacher in the family medicine residency program in Fort Collins, Colorado, and her colleagues audiotaped 300 visits to twenty-nine board-certified family physicians. As usual, the physicians greeted the patients and asked them why they had come to see them. How long do you think the physicians let the patient talk before interrupting to ask a second question? Two minutes? You're way off. One minute? Not even close.

These experienced physicians waited an average of just *eighteen seconds* before interrupting the patient. If you're tempted to think the physicians were speeding things up to save time and get to the point faster, consider this. The study found that, once interrupted, the patients never got back to describing fully the reason why they came to the doctor. As a result, the physicians actually missed a chance to get a complete grasp of the diagnosis and increased the patients' sense of dissatisfaction. The study was published in 1999 in the *Journal of the American Medical Association*.

That was a study of family physicians, arguably the mavens of gathering patients' information. If anything, the problem of interrupting patients is far worse in the ER.

How do you use silence as a technique for history-taking when you can't buy it in the ER? It's not easy, considering all the noise and distractions, but it's important we do our best to stop talking and just listen. Frequently, the easiest time to do this is close to the end of a shift, when there's less pressure to keep "moving the meat."

"It was a while ago," she continued. "Before I was married." She checked my reaction, misjudging what I assumed was a quizzical look on my face to be concern as to whether her husband was aware this had happened. "Steve knows."

I had indeed been thinking about what Jenny said but it didn't have to do with Steve. Something stuck in the throat, if not actual, could be psychological. I wanted to blurt, "Is there something you need to say? Something you find difficult getting out?" But I'm not a shrink, and she hadn't come to the ER for therapy, at least not consciously.

"Is anything troubling you?" I asked, deciding this was a safe and appropriate question for a doctor to pose in this circumstance.

She started nervously fingering a small silver cross that hung from a chain around her neck. "No," she replied.

I had a strong sense that Jenny was worried that God would punish her for the abortion—that she would lose the baby. But it was not my place to say that. Not directly. But perhaps I could skate around it.

"It's normal to be stressed during pregnancy," I said. "I also know many women who have had abortions, and many of them have been concerned that somehow it would be . . . harder, more difficult, to have a successful pregnancy once they conceived again."

I saw her nod as I said this.

"I just want to say that medically, if you've been checked out—"

"She's 100 percent healthy," Steve interjected. "We've had her checked top to bottom." I wondered if he was a mechanic, the way he said that.

"—if you're fine physically, there's no reason to worry about the baby or the birth," I said.

Jenny took this in, saying nothing for a few moments. "What about my throat?"

I told her I didn't think there was anything stuck there, that she likely had a slight irritation. "Some herbal tea with honey will help." I also suggested an over-the-counter tablet for heartburn.

After saying goodbye, I walked out of the room to write up my notes. Steve followed me.

"She thinks she's sinned," he said. "She's scared that . . ."

"If you can't reassure her, maybe some counselling," I said. "Or a progressive minister. Not one who will admonish her. One who will support her."

Steve shook my hand. "Thanks. You've been a real help."

They had come from their home to the ER seeking comfort. Or reassurance. As I went to the board to see what cases were left to mop up before my shift was over, I hoped I had given Jenny and Steve what they needed. Was it part of my job as an emergency doctor? I wasn't saving someone from cardiac arrest or some other life-threatening problem. But if my advice helped them deal better with what was one of the most important and vulnerable experiences in their life, then I had performed a healing function, which is what a doctor is supposed to do, in the ER or anywhere else. Right?

6:50 A.M.

One of the nurses came to my office to say there was an agitated patient, admitted a few hours earlier, whom she thought I should check on if I could. My replacement—the ER physician on the day shift—wasn't set to arrive for another ten minutes.

"If things were crazy I wouldn't bother you with him because I don't think there's anything medically wrong with him," she said. "I've put in a request for a social worker to see him as soon as she gets here later today. I think the guy just needs to be calmed down and reassured by seeing a doctor."

"Why is he here?"

"We're not exactly sure," the nurse said. "You see, he's deaf and he doesn't have any speech."

"Isn't there anyone on staff who can sign?"

"He doesn't sign."

"He doesn't sign?" This caught me totally by surprise. "How old is he?"

"About forty. He reads lips and then he writes out what he wants to say."

The nurse said this without any agitation in her voice. Like so many of the nurses, she was a compassionate person. Despite being tired at the end of a long shift, she didn't see this patient as an annoyance. In fact, the unusual aspect of the case probably boosted her energy, as it offered an interesting distraction from the typical ones she'd dealt with all night.

I assured her I'd be there as soon as I could.

She was a top-notch nurse, one who made my life easier rather than tougher. There are nurses who move patients along efficiently and others who don't. We say the latter are often suffering from "dyscopia," meaning they can't cope with their workload. Just as the nurses figure out if the ER doctor can move the meat, we also look to see what nurses are on duty and what their track record is.

The triage nurses are a patient's first point of entry to the ER. They have a tremendous responsibility to determine the seriousness of each person's situation. The physicians, and even more so the patients, rely on the triage nurses to prioritize the cases. Generally speaking, they do an amazing job. It's not easy managing an endless stream of sick people asking for or, in many cases, demanding help immediately. When all the beds inside the ER are full, they have to keep a special eye on patients in the waiting room who are there longer than the Canadian Trauma Acuity Scale (CTAS) says they should be.

It's not uncommon to have patients with belly pain wait several hours simply because there's no place to put them. Recently, Mount Sinai's ER became one of the first to try a cutting-edge practice that banks on the idea that not every patient with abdominal pain or a headache or vaginal bleeding (or a whole host of other conditions) needs to be placed on a stretcher. We converted a patient room inside the department into a "rapid assessment zone" or RAZ. Instead of one stretcher, the room contains six chairs, allowing ER docs to see up to six patients in a space previously meant for one. Anything to beef up our capacity to see people in a timely fashion.

If you wonder why some nurses develop a somewhat cold countenance as they deal with you in the triage process, you need to understand that after years of having people beg, threaten, lie, coerce and try every possible trick to get ahead in the line, they have learned that detachment is the only way to cope with the endless barrage of sick, hurt, angry, tired and frustrated people getting on their case.

Just as doctors don't like to have major cases come in at the end of a shift, the same is true for nurses. They don't want to hand over a large number of patients who are in the midst of being treated any more than we do.

How does this affect you? Try not to come in just as a shift is ending (as if you would know this, although you do now).

The deaf patient had a most nervous disposition. I placed myself in front of him so he could read my lips, a process I knew was by no means 100 percent accurate. My memory told me, from an article I'd once read, that some studies have determined that only about a third of English words can be lip-read.

Typically, lip-reading is accompanied by sign language and written communication. In this case, I found it hard to understand how an adult who said (through a note) that he had been deaf most of his life could not sign.

My patient said he had a headache. He was afraid he had a brain tumour. A physical examination didn't reveal anything, and I was able to reassure him.

He had a nervous demeanour and fidgeted non-stop. I asked if he took drugs. He said no and I believed him. His anxiety didn't resemble that of someone who did a lot of drugs. Nor did he accept when I offered him a tablet of lorazepam, a mild sedative, to calm him down. Most drug seekers say yes to any available drug.

It was difficult to communicate with him in any meaningful way, and I felt frustrated by my inability to get through to him. If I had seen him earlier in the shift I might have spent more time trying to find a way to connect. But it was late, and I was exhausted and somewhat impatient. I also wanted to ensure that I had cleared the board by the end of my shift.

A social worker would be around in a couple of hours, and she would be able to take more time with him. I saw nothing more that could be done unless the ultrasound revealed a medical problem. I'd see the results before leaving, which meant I could feel I wasn't dumping him on the next shift—unless a big problem arose, an unlikely outcome that I would deal with if it occurred.

7:00 A.M.

As I went to find my last patient, I walked past one of the custodial staff, who was cleaning the floor. A large, pleasant man, he shared with me a passion for the TV show *Lost*. He wanted to chat about the recent episodes, as we often did, but I had to take a rain check.

It's funny what goes through your mind and how fast it infiltrates your psyche. As the images of some *Lost* shows briefly flashed through my head I thought about an interview I had recently done for *White Coat, Black Art* with Dr. Rick Morris, a trauma physician at Foothills Hospital in Calgary. He had told me a couple of stories, one of which involved a man who had accidentally shot a crossbow arrow through his face and skull after consuming "about twenty rye and Cokes and a half-case of beer." Amazingly, the guy lived to tell about it.

Another was the type of story you might recount at a dinner party, thanks to the unusual nature of the outcome. It involved a man in his early nineties who had been out golfing during the day. At night, following a meal of "good ol' Alberta beef and potatoes," his wife noticed he was breathing funny during his sleep. She shook him, but he didn't wake up, so she called 911. The paramedics found his heart rate was 15 and his blood pressure very low. When they brought him to the ER it was assumed he would die.

The man was taken to the trauma bay and a central line was put into his neck. Morris inserted a temporary pacemaker into the line through a little wire. "Essentially we stick a needle and syringe into the internal jugular, a big vein in the neck," he said. "We take off the syringe and thread a wire through the needle, and then we put a catheter, which is a tube essentially, into the jugular vein and pull out the wire. Now you have the catheter sitting in the middle of the patient's jugular vein, which provides direct access to the heart. Then you thread a special pacemaker wire with a balloon at the tip through the catheter to the heart. Once you advance the catheter into the heart, you inflate the balloon and then you literally float the balloon into the heart. And this is mostly done blindly, without being able to see where you're going. Once the catheter is in, you just look at the monitor screen, aside from some momentary glimpses on a cineradiograph, or moving X-ray."

They were completing the most delicate part of the procedure, the moment when the leading edge of the pacemaker wire contained in the balloon touched the inside of the man's left ventricle, a part of his heart. As soon as it made contact, "He sat bolt upright with this thing hanging out of his neck, saying, 'What the hell? Where am I? What's going on? I was just in my bedroom,'" said Morris. "It was like the Lazarus effect. The guy was dying and within literally five seconds he was walking, talking, telling me about his dinner and couldn't believe he was in the hospital."

In hindsight, I wonder if Morris's second story had flitted through my mind because I was worried about what kind of condition my next patient was in. I hoped that whatever it was it would have a similarly good outcome.

Fran was about sixty and not in good physical shape. She was overweight and had large, pendulous breasts. Fran lived alone and had come in by taxi after feeling a shortness of breath a few hours earlier. I noticed her legs were swollen and retaining water. She told me she had had bypass surgery a year or so ago, but until tonight she had thought her heart was working fine. She also said she was on a beta blocker, a common remedy for someone with a heart condition. The drug, which goes under numerous brand names, reduces heart rate and blood pressure, and thus can help protect the heart.

As I spoke with her it was obvious she was scared, which was not surprising. I asked her several questions.

"How many pillows do you sleep with?" I asked this because patients with heart failure tend to have blood backing up into their lungs. They sleep more upright to allow the blood to pool in the lower part of their lungs, enabling the upper parts of the lungs to do a better job of taking in oxygen.

"Two."

"Do you weigh yourself every day?" If she was gaining weight rapidly, that would be a sign of water retention, a telltale symptom of heart failure.

"Yes."

I checked her chest with my stethoscope and could hear a slight crackling sound, a sure indication of water in the lungs. With each moment, it was getting clearer that my patient had congestive heart failure. I needed to order a chest X-ray and do some blood tests to rule out a heart attack. I also ordered an arterial blood gas to check for hypoxia, a sign of respiratory distress.

I sighed to myself. There was no way I was going to hand this patient over. She'd waited far too long to see me. I felt bad she'd waited so long. Call it conscientiousness or call it guilt, but I was determined to make sure she was properly looked after.

"Will I be okay?" Fran asked.

"I'm pretty sure you will," I said, smiling and patting her on the shoulder.

"You doing any exercise?" I asked as I was leaving.

"Yeah."

"Really?"

"No. But I will. I will."

I'd heard that promise many times. Sometimes it was true and often it wasn't. I wished Fran well. I went to the board to make sure there were no patients I'd forgotten to see. This happens more times than many of us choose to admit. There's nothing more embarrassing to me than having agreed to see a patient but not remembering to do so. Fortunately, there were none.

7:10 A.M.

My replacement walked in with a sheepish smile and an apology for being ten minutes late. The code among ER physicians is that ten minutes late is trivial. Twenty minutes late is considered rude. Once you're thirty minutes late and counting, the doctor still on duty—not to mention the nurses—begin to wonder whether you're going to show up.

"Do you remember" isn't the only triplet of words an ER physician never wants to hear. "Where are you?"—meaning you're scheduled to work and nowhere to be found—ranks up there with phrases that make your pulse race and a pit form in your gut.

Once every few years, while I'm getting a haircut or taking a nap, I get a call from the ER asking if I'm aware that I'm supposed to be on duty. I gather my things and race to the hospital, cursing and muttering all the way, while trying to get into the frame of mind of an ER physician. Fortunately, I don't drink much alcohol, and so that's unlikely to interfere with my competence on short notice.

The end of a night shift is a wonderful time for me. I feel this immense relief that the next critically ill patient who bursts through the swinging doors won't be my responsibility. It feels as if the treadmill I've been running on all night has stopped. No longer do I have to see new patients. Now I only have to figure out what to do with the ones I've already seen.

As my colleague took over, I felt euphoric. This was no accident. A number of recent studies have found that pulling an all-nighter raises the mood of up to 60 percent of people suffering from depression. But the effect is only temporary. Still, I always look forward to that predictable buzz following a night shift. The other nice thing about the end of my shift is that I have time to chat with fellow staff and patients. The relentless pace of emergency medicine makes it difficult to do so until my shift is over.

I used to laugh when I watched the doctors on TV shows like *ER* hand patients over to their colleagues before going home. They would hand off the most outrageous tasks. For instance, they'd walk out saying a patient had suspected meningitis and would the colleague mind doing a lumbar puncture (also known as a spinal tap) to rule it out. A lumbar puncture takes thirty to forty-five minutes. It can be painful, and you have to explain to the patient the purpose of the test, how it feels to get it done, and the risks. The test is done with mask, surgical drape, gown and gloves. You need a minimum of one doctor and one nurse, and often a second nurse, to get it done.

Believe me, conscientious ER docs never leave an LP to be done by a colleague—unless of course they work on TV instead of in the real world.

9:00 A.M.

This shift, I got lucky. I didn't have to hand over a single patient to my colleague. In other words, I was able to discharge patients or refer them to a consultant. I know my colleague was pleased. Peering out into the waiting room, I could see a line of five patients waiting to be triaged. Looking at a monitor located above a sink in the main nursing area, I could see that three crews of paramedics were on their way bearing one CTAS 2 and two CTAS 3 patients. I felt for my colleague. He was in for a long day.

I visited Sophia one more time to see how she was doing. She was like a new woman. Her breathing was no longer laboured, and the rate had dropped to a normal sixteen breaths a minute. No longer did she look as if she needed to be put on a ventilator. She was awake enough to be complaining about pain from her chest tube and from her cancer.

As John Ross, my friend and colleague from QEII Health Sciences Centre in Halifax, would say, it's easy to put the tube down the throat and put a patient on a ventilator. My knowledge and experience had led me away from the knee-jerk response to give Sophia what she needed. I've heard experienced surgeons say that the toughest surgical decision is the one *not* to operate. It was one of those special moments when I inspired the residents to believe in me. My professional satisfaction was tempered by the certain knowledge that, sooner or later, Sophia would succumb to the awful disease that was destroying her body.

Just not today.

I headed out the sliding doors of the ER and into the bracing cold of a mid-winter morning. The icy wind felt good against my face. Most nights, I'm happy if I take care of my patients and nothing bad happens. This was a rare shift in which I dwelled for a moment on still being able to make a difference in someone's life.

I headed for the subway, which would leave me a short walk from home. There are times when I fall asleep on the train. I'm glad I don't have a car at my disposal.

I boarded the subway train that runs south several stations before looping north with a great screeching sound that always bothers my sensitive ears. I shivered a bit. Each year, as I get older, the damp winter of the city bothers me even more. It's in those moments following a shift, when the euphoria has begun to pass, that another kind of coldness touches my heart. It's a reality that few of my ER colleagues talk about but many feel.

"Do you remember?" That's the question I hope—despite all evidence to the contrary—that I'll never hear again. Of course I will; probably it will happen at a moment when I've let down my guard and deluded myself into believing that I've grown beyond human frailty and weakness.

Of course I remember. I remember each and every patient. They visit me during my waking life. And they come to me in my dreams—even the ones I have during the day when I sleep while others are awake.

I'd be lying if I said I always feel pride and pleasure for a job well done. Ours is a calling in which praise is taken with a dose of skepticism. As I walked home from the subway station, tired to my bones, I felt instead relief: that I didn't forget to order a test or check on a CT scan; that I didn't send someone home whom I should have admitted; that I didn't screw up.

At least until my next shift.